# Make Weight Smart

## The Ketogenic Approach for Boxers

Andy Hodges

Boxing Lab Academy Publications

laboratoryboxing@gmail.com

## DEDICATION

To fighters, coaches, and everyone who believes that making weight should be guided by structure, discipline, and understanding — not by methods that sacrifice health and destroy performance.

CONTENTS

## ACKNOWLEDGEMENTS

I would like to thank the tutors on my England Boxing Level 3 Senior Coach course (Cohort 2024/2025), led by head tutor Ivan, along with Laura, Alan, Adam, Steve, and John, for their guidance, high standards, and for pushing me beyond my comfort zone.

The ketogenic diet was the focus of my Level 3 project, where I set out to answer a simple question – can it actually work for boxers, and if so, how do you apply it properly without compromising performance?

That work became the foundation for this book. Their emphasis on understanding, structure, and doing things properly shaped the approach taken here.

This book is built on that process – helping boxers make weight smarter, stay strong, and perform at their best.

I would also like to thank my friend Carly for her support in editing this book and helping give it its final shape. Her patience, feedback, and attention to detail throughout the process were sincerely appreciated.

## FOREWORD

*Make Weight Smarter, Not Harder*

Boxing teaches more than how to throw a punch. It teaches control – discipline, respect, patience, and courage – not just over your opponent, but over yourself. But there's one part of the sport where that control often disappears: making weight.

This book is not about shortcuts or miracle diets. It's about structure, awareness, and control. It's about understanding how your body works so that making weight becomes part of your training, not something you fear at the end of it.

The approach in this book uses ketogenic principles, not because they are trendy, but because when applied correctly, they can be a powerful tool. A way to fuel smarter, reduce body fat without losing strength, and stay consistent throughout camp. This is not about following a diet blindly. It's about understanding how your body uses fuel and using that knowledge to stay in control.

There is a simple reason for writing this book. Boxing needs a practical, fight-focused guide but hasn't had one. Most nutrition advice comes from endurance sports, bodybuilding, or clinical settings. But boxing is different. The timelines are tighter, the pressure around the scale is higher, and the culture around weight cutting is still built on outdated habits. Fighters don't need theory. They need something that fits real training, real camps, and real fight week pressure. Based on both personal experience and a review of research, I believe that a ketogenic approach to nutrition can offer boxers the way forward that they need.

Inside, you'll find a full twelve-round system that takes you from understanding food and fuel, through adaptation and hydration, to fight week strategy, and long-term control. Each part builds on the next, because performance doesn't come from one decision. It comes from a system.

The system proposed here is evidence based and respects the expertise of health professionals. Before making any major changes, speak to a qualified professional such as a GP, sports dietitian, or registered nutritionist. If you are under eighteen, on medication, or managing a medical condition, this is essential. Women boxers should also consult an appropriate health professional before deciding whether to try the ketogenic approach, as it can impact on the hormonal balance required for women's reproductive and metabolic health. Making weight should never come at the cost of your health.

The mission of Boxing Lab Academy is simple. Make health education part of training. When you understand your body, you stop fearing the scale. You walk into competition focused, fuelled, and ready to perform, not recover.

If this book helps you move from guessing to planning, from cutting weight to controlling it, then it has done its job. Train smart. Respect your body. Stay in control.

*Andy Hodges – Boxing Lab Academy*

# ROUND 1

# RETHINK THE CUT

## *Why Old-School Weight Drops Fail*

In boxing, every kilogram matters. Weight divisions exist for a reason: to create a fair playing field. But the way fighters have traditionally made weight has always been a gamble – one where everything they've worked for is put on the line before the fight even begins.

Because "making weight" doesn't happen under the lights. It happens in the days before, behind closed doors – when no one's watching.

### 1.1 THE COST OF OLD-SCHOOL CUTTING

For decades, making weight in boxing has been treated like a test of suffering. A badge of honour. Early mornings in a silent gym. Bin bags pulled tight. Heat building underneath. Sweat running down your back while the air around you feels heavy and still. You move, not to get better – but just to lose more.. Food and even water become things you earn, not things you rely on. Time slows down, and everything starts to revolve around one thing. The number on the scale. It stops being about the opponent. It stops being about the fight. The scales become the opponent.

I remember standing on the scale, completely drained, waiting for the number to settle. For a second, nothing else matters. Then it lands – and there it is. Relief. You made it. But it's a hollow kind of victory.

Yes, it works. The weight comes down.

But what comes next is harder to admit.

The lack of energy. The heaviness in your body. The split-second reactions that just aren't there. The quiet doubt that creeps in, even if you try to ignore it. You tell yourself you're ready – but deep down, you know something's missing. *I made weight.* But I didn't get better. *I made weight.* But I wasn't at my best. *I made weight* – but I was chasing the scale instead of chasing the win.

That was the system. That was how it was done. You didn't question it, because no one did. It was just part of the sport. Part of proving you were tough enough. But tradition isn't truth. It isn't common sense. It isn't safety. And it definitely isn't a guarantee of winning. What it does guarantee is this: you can do everything you were taught, hit the number exactly as expected – and still lose the fight before you ever step into the ring.

Now we know better.

When you strip water from the body, through restricting fluids or through excessive perspiration, you're not just losing weight – you're disrupting everything that keeps you performing.

Blood volume drops. The heart must work harder. Muscles don't contract as efficiently. What should feel sharp starts to feel heavy. Strength fades. Punches that should snap, don't. Reactions slow – fractions of a second, but enough to matter. Coordination dips. Timing slips. And the brain feels it too.

Research has shown that even a 2% drop in body water can impair cognitive performance, reaction time, and decision-making – exactly the things a fighter relies on under pressure. Discipline. But it doesn't feel like discipline. Recovery drags. Sleep is off. The nervous system stays under pressure, never fully switching off. Stress hormones stay elevated. The body holds on, instead of rebuilding. You can rehydrate. You can eat again. But physiology doesn't reset overnight. The system needs time – and in boxing, time is the one thing you don't have between weigh-in and fight night.

And the weight? It comes back. Glycogen stores refill. Water follows. Sometimes quickly. Sometimes unevenly. So you do it all again. That's not discipline. That's damage.

For years, fighters had to be tough just to survive bad weight cuts. Tough enough to ignore the signals. Tough enough to accept feeling flat, slow, and off – and still step into the ring like nothing was wrong. But toughness is never the goal. Performance is.

Performance improves when weight is managed properly – early, consistently, and with structure. Not in the final days through extremes, but from the start through control. Fuel the body properly, and energy systems work the way they're supposed to. Hydrate properly, and the brain and body stay connected. Recover properly, and adaptation actually happens. With real food. Proper hydration. Smart recovery.

This book isn't here to criticise the past. It's here to improve the future. Because when you understand why nutrition matters, discipline changes. It's no longer punishment. It becomes purpose. We're not eating less. We're eating better.

*Panic cutting vs Professional Preparation*

| PANIC CUTTING | PROFESSIONAL PREPARATION |
| --- | --- |
| Skips meals to drop weight fast | **Balances calories and nutrients gradually** |
| Trains in sweat suits to lose water | **Trains normally while monitoring hydration** |
| Drastically cuts carbs or salt | **Adjusts nutrition progressively based on load** |
| Ignores recovery | **Tracks sleep, rest, and fatigue** |
| Weighs daily and panics | **Logs weekly trends with coach review** |

***Coach's Insight:*** *Most fighters don't lose because of skill – they lose because they're drained before the fight starts.*

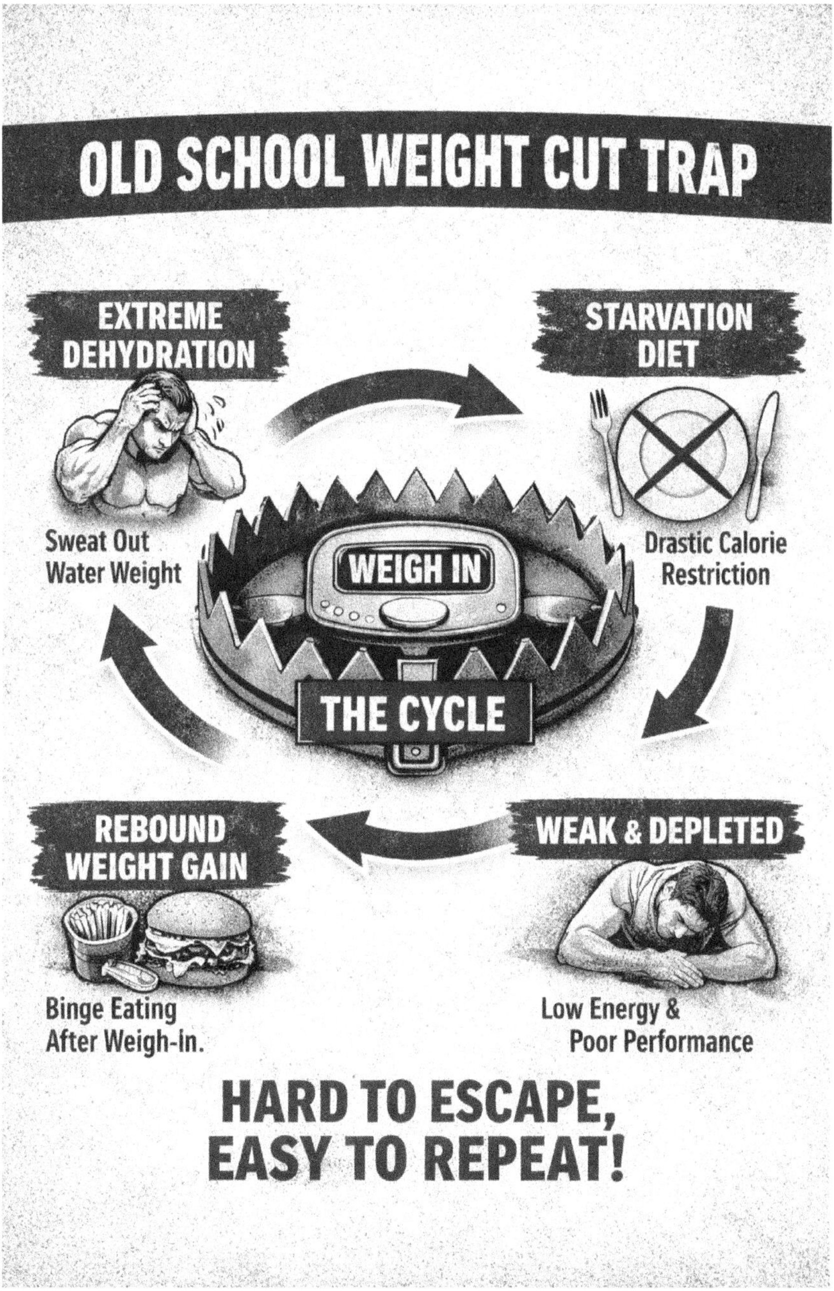
OLD SCHOOL WEIGHT CUT TRAP
EXTREME DEHYDRATION
STARVATION DIET
Sweat Out Water Weight
WEIGH IN
Drastic Calorie Restriction
THE CYCLE
REBOUND WEIGHT GAIN
WEAK & DEPLETED
Binge Eating After Weigh-In.
Low Energy & Poor Performance
HARD TO ESCAPE, EASY TO REPEAT!

## 1.2 FROM TRADITION TO UNDERSTANDING

Old-school boxing gyms built toughness. There's no denying that.

Early mornings. Repetition. Sweat on the floor. Round after round, doing the same things until they became automatic. You learned to push through fatigue. To keep going when your body said stop. That's always been part of the sport. But toughness without understanding comes at a cost.

It shows up later. In burnout. In injuries that don't fully heal. In fighters who train hard – but stop improving. The effort is there, but something's missing. Because effort alone isn't enough. Modern boxing still values discipline. That hasn't changed. But now, discipline is paired with understanding. Training, nutrition, and recovery aren't separate anymore. They work together.

Each one supporting the other. Or holding it back. Fuel isn't optional. Hydration isn't optional. Recovery isn't optional. They are part of performance. Because every session you do depends on how well your body is supported. Not just how hard you push – but how well you can repeat it, recover from it, and build on it. That's where the shift happens.

That's the evolution of the sport. Not replacing tradition – but refining it. Keeping the grit. Keeping the discipline. But adding understanding. Because when you combine both, you don't just protect your health – you improve your performance where it matters most. Inside the ring.

*Safe Weight-Making vs Old Habits*

| OLD SCHOOL | MODERN APPROACH |
| --- | --- |
| STARVE | **PLAN** |
| SWEAT | **CONTROL** |
| GUESS | **MONITOR** |
| PANIC | **EXECUTE** |

Old habits chase weight. Smart systems control it.

***Coach's Insight:*** *Respect the old school – but don't copy it blindly. Combine hard work with understanding.*

## 1.3 DISCIPLINE REDEFINED

Real discipline shows up long before fight week.

It is not built in the final few days, when pressure is high and mistakes are harder to fix. It is built earlier – through habits that are repeated consistently and without drama.

In boxing, discipline means planning ahead. It means knowing where your weight is, how your energy feels, and whether your recovery is supporting the work you are doing. It means paying attention instead of avoiding the problem and hoping it sorts itself out later.

That is what creates control.

When habits are consistent, the body becomes more predictable. When the body becomes more predictable, performance becomes more reliable. And when performance becomes more reliable, confidence grows with it.

This is why nutrition should be treated as part of training. Not as punishment. Not as a separate problem to deal with later. Just another part of the job that needs to be done properly.

Before changing anything drastically, start with the basics: clearly understand what you are doing and why, plan early, monitor regularly, recover properly, and stay consistent. That is what real discipline looks like in practice.

> ***Coach's Insight:*** *Discipline is not what you do when panic starts. It is what you repeat early enough to stop panic happening at all.*

## 1.4 LEARNING THE BODY'S LANGUAGE

Every phase of training places a different demand on the body.

Technical sessions require focus and precision. Conditioning blocks require sustained effort. Fight week requires control – managing weight while maintaining strength, speed, and clarity.

To handle this properly, a boxer needs more than discipline. They need awareness.

The body is constantly giving feedback. Energy levels, hunger, recovery, sleep quality, hydration – all of these are signals. When those signals are ignored, decisions become reactive. When they are understood, decisions become controlled.

A drop in energy is not always a sign to push harder. Sometimes it is a sign that fuel is low. Constant hunger is not always a lack of discipline. It can be a sign that structure is missing. Poor recovery is not just fatigue. It may reflect hydration, nutrition, or workload that is not balanced correctly.

This is where many boxers go wrong. They react emotionally instead of reading what is actually happening. They eat less when energy drops. They train harder when fatigue builds. They try to force results instead of adjusting the system.

Learning the body's language changes that.

Instead of reacting, the boxer starts responding. Adjustments become smaller, earlier, and more effective. Training becomes more consistent. Energy becomes more predictable. Recovery becomes part of the process, not something that is constantly chased.

Over time, this builds confidence. Not from guessing, but from understanding what the body is telling you and knowing how to act on it.

---

***Coach's Insight:*** *Your body always gives feedback. The difference is whether you ignore it – or use it.*

---

**SUMMARY:** ***The shift begins***

Making weight is no longer about last-minute effort. It is about planning early, managing consistently, and avoiding extremes.

Old habits rely on panic. A structured approach replaces that with control.

When weight is managed properly from the start, the process becomes more predictable. Training quality improves, recovery is more consistent, and fight week becomes execution instead of survival.

The key shift is simple: stop reacting late, and start managing early.

Next, we look at how food supports that process – and why getting it wrong creates many of the problems boxers face.

# ROUND 2

# THE REAL ROLE OF FOOD

## *Fuel, Not the Enemy*

In boxing, food is often treated like the enemy. Fighters try to eat as little as possible – especially when a fight is coming up. On the surface, it looks like discipline. It looks like control. But it isn't. Because what usually follows is low energy, slower recovery, and a body that doesn't respond the way it should.

The problem was never food. The problem is how food is understood. Food supports everything you do in training. Food needs to stop being something you "cut." It has to become something you *use*. As important as gloves. As important as pads. As important as the rounds themselves. You will feel the difference. You can push harder without breaking down. You stay sharper for longer. You recover more quickly between sessions. Training starts to build – not just take. Weight stops being a last-minute problem. When it's managed early, with consistency and structure, fight week feels different. No panic. No desperation. Just execution. You step on the scale ready – not drained.

This round focuses on achieving this..

Not by eating less – but by understanding how to fuel properly, build structure, and stay in control of body weight without constant restriction.

## 2.1 THE BINGE–RESTRICT CYCLE

This is one of the most common patterns in boxing – and one of the most damaging.

A boxer wants to make weight. So they start by cutting food. Meals get smaller. Snacks disappear. Sometimes entire meals are skipped. At first, it feels like control. The weight might drop quickly. The scale starts moving in the right direction.

But underneath that, something else is happening. Energy drops. Hunger increases. Cravings get stronger. The body is not designed to perform well when it is under-fuelled. It starts pushing back. When food intake drops too low, the body responds by increasing hunger signals and reducing energy output. This is a normal biological response – not a lack of discipline.

The body is trying to protect itself. And sooner or later, the restriction breaks. The boxer eats more than planned. Sometimes a little more. Sometimes a lot more. It might be late at night. It might be after a hard session. It might come from feeling exhausted, frustrated, or simply too hungry to ignore. This is the binge.

After that comes the reaction: Guilt. Panic. The feeling that everything has been undone. So the next day, the boxer goes even harder: Eat less. Cut more. Train harder. And the cycle repeats. This is the binge–restrict cycle.

***Coach's Insight:*** *If you're constantly overeating after restricting, it's a bad system. Fix the system.*

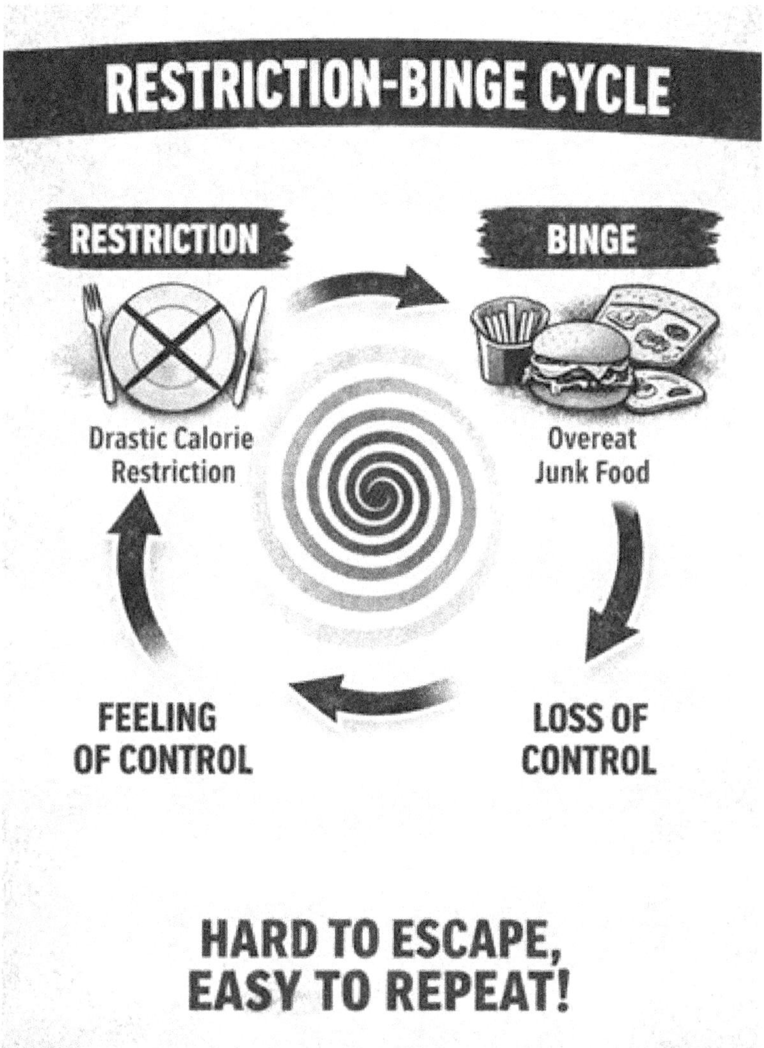

## 2.2 WHY "EATING LESS" DOESN'T WORK

At first, eating less feels like the obvious answer. If weight needs to go down, just reduce food. Simple. And in the short term, it works. The scale drops. The boxer feels lighter. There's a sense of progress.

But the body doesn't just lose weight – it reacts. When food intake drops too low, the body shifts into a protective mode. It doesn't understand "making weight." It understands survival. So it starts adjusting.

Energy availability drops, and the body begins to conserve fuel instead of using it freely. Training output decreases, and recovery slows. Hormonal signals also change. Hunger increases. So do feelings of stress. . Concentration drops but relaxation becomes difficult. This isn't lack of discipline – it's the body trying to restore balance.

At the same time, the body becomes more efficient – but not in a good way. It reduces how much energy it uses.

Daily movement drops without you noticing.

Recovery becomes slower. So even though you're eating less, fat loss can slow down – or stop completely.

And while this is happening, pressure builds. Cravings increase, and training starts to feel harder than it should. Eventually, the system breaks – and the binge–restrict cycle returns. This is why "just eating less" doesn't work long-term. Because the goal isn't just to lose weight – it's to train, recover, and perform properly. And that requires energy.

The better question is not: "How can I eat less?" It's: "How can I fuel properly while staying in control of my weight?" That's where real progress starts.

This doesn't mean fasting can't be used. The difference is simple – random restriction breaks performance, while structured fasting is planned, controlled, and used with purpose. One is reactive. The other is strategic.

We'll come back to that later.

> ***Coach's Insight:*** *You can't train like a fighter and eat like you're inactive. Low fuel always shows up in performance.*

## 2.3 FOOD AS FUEL

Every action in boxing depends on energy.

Not just punching and moving – but timing, reactions, decision-making, and the ability to stay sharp under pressure. These are not just skills. They are supported by how well the body is fuelled.

When energy is available, everything works the way it should. Combinations flow. Movement feels lighter. Reactions stay quick, even as fatigue builds. You can maintain output across rounds and recover more effectively between efforts.

When energy is not supported properly, the drop is noticeable.

Timing starts to slip. Reactions slow slightly. Combinations feel heavier. It is not always obvious at first, but over time it shows – especially in longer sessions or under pressure.

This is where many boxers misunderstand performance. They separate training from nutrition, as if effort alone is enough. But training increases demand. Nutrition is what supports that demand.

If the body is not fuelled correctly, it cannot produce the same level of output – no matter how motivated the boxer is.

Food provides three key things:

- ✓ Energy to train and perform
- ✓ Materials to recover and rebuild
- ✓ Support for the brain and nervous system

Without that, performance is limited – not just physically, but mentally as well.

At the same time, quality matters.

Whole, consistent food sources tend to support stable energy and better recovery. Poor-quality or inconsistent intake often leads to fluctuations – short periods of feeling good, followed by drops in energy and focus.

This is not about eating more or less. It is about matching intake to the demands of training.

When food is used properly, it becomes a tool that supports performance – not something that interferes with it.

> ***Coach's Insight:*** *Performance doesn't just come from how hard you train. It comes from how well your body is supported to do that work.*

## 2.4 STRUCTURE OVER GUESSWORK

One of the biggest mistakes boxers make with nutrition is relying on guesswork. Eating randomly. Skipping meals. Eating based on mood, hunger, or stress. Some days they eat very little. Other days, far more than planned. There's no consistency behind it – no system. And without structure, there is no control.

This is where problems start to build. Energy becomes unpredictable. One session feels sharp, the next feels flat. Recovery doesn't follow a pattern. Body weight moves up and down without any clear reason.

The boxer ends up reacting instead of planning. "I'll eat less today." "I'll train harder tomorrow." "I'll fix it next week."

But nothing really gets fixed – because there is no foundation behind it.

The body performs best when energy intake is consistent. When meals are regular and predictable, the system becomes more stable. Energy doesn't spike and crash as much. Training becomes more repeatable. Recovery starts to support the work instead of holding it back.

Structure doesn't mean strict dieting or extreme rules.

It means having a clear, consistent way of eating that supports your training. It means regular meals. A balanced intake. A routine that fits around your sessions instead of working against them.

When that structure is in place, things begin to settle.

Decisions become easier. You're not constantly reacting to how you feel in the moment. You're following a system that has a purpose behind it.

And that system doesn't need to be complicated.

In fact, the simpler it is, the better. Consistency beats intensity – in training and in nutrition. It's not what you do once that matters. It's what you repeat.

Structure creates consistency. Consistency creates control.

*Weekly Weight and Wellness Log - Template*

| WEEK | BODY WEIGHT (kg) | ENERGY (1-5) | SLEEP (hrs) | NOTES |
|---|---|---|---|---|
| 1 | | | | |
| 2 | | | | |
| 3 | | | | |
| 4 | | | | |
| 5 | | | | |

Regular tracking builds awareness. It also teaches responsibility – a key skill in both sport and life.

***Coach's Insight:*** *What you do occasionally doesn't matter. What you do consistently decides your performance.*

## 2.5 WHAT HAPPENS WHEN FOOD IS CONTROLLED

When food is managed properly, the changes are not dramatic overnight – but they are clear.

The first thing that improves is consistency.

Energy becomes more stable across the day. Sessions feel more predictable. Instead of sharp highs and sudden drops, output becomes easier to maintain from start to finish.

Training quality follows.

You can hold pace more effectively, stay sharper under fatigue, and complete sessions without the same drop-off in performance. Not because you are doing more, but because the body is better supported to do the work.

Recovery also becomes more reliable.

Between sessions, the body has what it needs to repair and reset. Fatigue does not carry over in the same way, and you are more prepared for the next session instead of constantly catching up.

Hunger becomes easier to manage.

Instead of constant cravings or sudden urges to eat, appetite follows a more predictable pattern. This removes a lot of the emotional response around food and makes decisions simpler.

Body weight becomes more controlled.

Rather than large fluctuations, changes happen gradually. This reduces pressure and removes the need for extreme adjustments later on.

At the same time, stress around food begins to drop.

You are no longer reacting to every meal or every change on the scale. You are following a system that gives you direction and control.

This is the difference between guessing and managing.

It does not mean everything becomes perfect. There will still be adjustments to make. But the process becomes clearer, more stable, and easier to handle.

That is what most boxers are actually aiming for – not just to be lighter, but to perform better with less disruption.

***Coach's Insight:*** *When your food is under control, everything else becomes easier – training, recovery, and decision-making.*

**SUMMARY:** ***From restriction to control***

Most boxers don't struggle because they lack discipline.

They struggle because they misunderstand food. Eating less, skipping meals, or constantly restricting intake might feel like control – but it usually leads to the opposite. Unstable energy. Poor training. Inconsistent weight. Frustration around food. The binge–restrict cycle is not a personal failure. It's a predictable response to under-fuelling the body. To move forward, the approach has to change.

When you start treating it that way, everything begins to stabilise. Structure replaces guesswork. Control replaces reaction.

You stop chasing short-term results and start building a system that supports performance. When that system is in place, recovery improves, body weight becomes more predictable. And just as important, your relationship with food becomes simpler and more controlled.

At this stage, you don't need complexity. You need understanding. You need direction. Because once food stops being something you fight against, it becomes one of your biggest advantages in the ring.

Up to this point, we've focused on behaviour and structure. Next, it's time to understand what's happening inside the body – and how energy is actually produced.

# ROUND 3

# MACRONUTRIENTS

## *The Building Blocks*

All food is made up of three main components:

- Protein
- Fats
- Carbohydrates

These are called macronutrients. They are not just numbers on a meal plan. Each one has a specific role in how your body performs, recovers, and manages weight. Each macronutrient influences how the body produces energy at a cellular level. This affects not just how you feel, but how you perform under fatigue, how you recover between sessions, and how well you maintain output over time.

**Protein** is used to repair and rebuild the body. Every hard session creates stress and damage that needs to be recovered from. Without enough protein, recovery is slower and performance suffers.

**Fats** support overall health and long-term energy. They play a key role in hormone function, including those that affect recovery, strength, and wellbeing.

**Carbohydrates** provide quick, accessible energy. They are the main fuel for high-intensity efforts – fast combinations, sharp reactions, and explosive work.

A boxer doesn't just need less food or more food. They need the right balance of these three. This is where many mistakes happen. Some cut carbohydrates too aggressively. Some avoid fats completely. Some don't eat enough protein to recover properly. Without understanding these basics, it's easy to:

- Lose muscle instead of fat
- Feel low on energy
- Struggle in training
- Make weight harder instead of easier

Getting this balance wrong doesn't just affect body weight. It affects performance. At this stage, you don't need to overcomplicate it. Just understand this: Your body runs on a combination of these three nutrients. And how you balance them will directly impact how you train and perform.

We will break each of them down properly later in the book. For now, the key message is simple: It's not just about how much you eat. It's about what your food is made of.

***Coach's Insight:*** *It's not just about eating less – it's about eating right. The balance of your food matters as much as the amount.*

## 3.1 PROTEIN – REPAIR AND STRENGTH

Protein is what builds the body and protects the boxer.

Every session creates stress on the body. Pads, sparring, conditioning – all of it breaks tissue down. That's normal. But progress doesn't happen during training. It happens when the body builds and repairs itself. And that process depends on protein.

Protein provides amino acids – the building blocks the body uses to build and repair all its tissues, particularly muscle, to increase or maintain strength, and to adapt to training. Without enough protein, conditioning stops, recovery slows down. Fatigue builds. Performance becomes inconsistent.

During a weight cut, this becomes even more important. When calories drop, the body looks for energy. When carbohydrates are low, the body will eventually start to burn fat – this is central to the ketogenic approach described in this book -- but first it may start to burn protein. In protein rich diet, this protein will be found in dietary intake, and the body will then move on to burning fat, but if the diet is low on protein, the body may start to burn the protein that makes up muscle. This will result in:

- Loss of strength
- Reduced power
- Slower metabolism
- Worse performance

This is one of the biggest mistakes boxers make. They eat less – including protein – and end up lighter, but weaker.

Protein is not what you cut. It's what you protect. It helps maintain lean muscle, which keeps metabolism higher and supports performance.

Protein needs to stay consistent – not excessive, but not low. Balance matters. Because in boxing, it's not just about losing weight. It's about losing the right weight – without losing what makes you dangerous.

---

***Coach's Insight:*** *You don't build strength in the session – you build it in recovery. Protein is what makes that happen.*

---

## 3.2 CARBOHYDRATES – THE STANDARD FUEL

Throughout human history, people have relied on different food sources, depending on season, climate, geography, and availability. Carbohydrates from fruits, berries, roots, and later grains were accessible depending on seasonal availability.

Sugars found in berries and fruit, along with starches from grains and roots, are broken down by the body into glucose – its most basic and readily available energy fuel.

Highly processed carbohydrates – particularly sugars – can be converted very quickly to glucose. An "energy drink" based on white sugar or even neat glucose will hit the bloodstream almost immediately and provide an intense burst of energy – followed by a rapid crash.

Less processed carbohydrates, such as whole grains, are converted more slowly and produce a glucose-releasing compound called glycogen, which is stored in the tissues. These provide a rather more prolonged source of energy but one which can still abruptly plummet when the store runs out – the experience often called "hitting the wall".

## 3.3 THE ROLE OF CARBOHYDRATES

Carbohydrates are often the most misunderstood part of a boxer's diet. Some rely on them too much. Others try to remove them completely. The truth sits in the middle. Carbohydrates are the body's quickest source of energy. They are especially useful for:

- ✓ High-intensity training
- ✓ Explosive combinations
- ✓ Sprint work
- ✓ Hard sparring sessions

This is why boxers traditionally rely on them. They provide fast fuel. But they also come with limitations. Carbohydrates are stored in the body as glycogen – and that storage is limited. Once it runs out, energy drops quickly. Every boxer knows what it feels like to "run out of gas."

It's that moment when the body feels heavy, reactions slow, and the mind struggles to stay sharp – even if the fitness is there.

This doesn't mean carbohydrates are bad – it means their role needs to be understood and controlled.

The mistake is to rely on them constantly. This creates:

- Energy spikes and crashes
- Increased hunger
- Less control over body weight

The goal is not to fear carbohydrates. And it's not to depend on them blindly. The goal is to use them with purpose. To match them to the demands of training. To support performance – without losing control of energy or weight. Because in boxing, the best results come from understanding your fuel – not just following habits.

---

***Coach's Insight:*** *Carbs aren't the problem – using them without purpose is.*

---

## 3.4 FATS – A BUILDING BLOCK AND MORE

Fat is also essential for health. It supports hormone functions – including those linked to recovery, strength, and overall performance. It supports the brain and nervous system – which are critical for focus, timing, and decision-making in the ring. And it helps regulate hunger. Meals that include enough fat tend to keep you full for longer, reducing cravings and making it easier to stay consistent with your nutrition. This is one of the reasons why some boxers feel more in control when using a structured higher-fat approach. But not all fats are equal. The focus should be on quality sources:

- ✓ Oily fish (salmon, sardines, mackerel)
- ✓ Eggs
- ✓ Avocados
- ✓ Butter
- ✓ Olive oil
- ✓ Nuts and seeds

These provide both energy and important nutrients that support performance and recovery. Highly processed fats, on the other hand, offer little benefit and should be limited. Foods high in unhelpful processed fats include:

- Packaged snacks such as crisps and biscuits
- Commercial baked cakes and pastries
- Fast food and frozen meals
- Reconstituted meat such as hot-dogs and sausages
- Ice cream, flavoured yogurt, and processed cheese

These are the fats which contribute least to the positive functions of fat, and most to the storage of unwanted fat in the body.

## 3.5 CUTTING WEIGHT BY MANAGING FUEL

As described above, the body's standard "fuel" is glucose, which is usually derived from carbohydrates. When there is insufficient glucose from carbohydrates, the body can also create glucose by breaking down protein, and to a lesser extent fat. If the body is starved, it will draw instead on the body's own tissues, muscle and fat.

This is the basis for standard weight-loss diets. Just starve the body of fuel, and weight loss will result. This approach, rigorously and consistently applied over a long period – will indeed have this result. However, as discussed in the previous chapter, losing weight by just cutting food triggers reactions that undermine this outcome.

Deprived of fuel, the body fights back. And it does so in ways which are particularly damaging for an athlete. Energy levels drop, leading to crashes which impact on training and performance. The body may start to break down dietary protein or even its own muscle to create glucose, resulting in a loss of muscle strength and delays in muscle repair. Conditioning becomes impossible. With insufficient fuel, hunger increases, and cravings lead to bingeing. This sort of dieting can cut weight in the short term, but for most athletes it doesn't work long term.

The ketogenic diet depends on a different approach. The body has a different way of fuelling itself, which standard diets don't tap into. Under the right conditions, the body can be taught to move from burning glucose from carbohydrates as its primary fuel to burning molecules called *ketones* which are created by directly breaking down fat. This is the basis of the ketogenic approach, and its effect on the body is very different.

The ketogenic approach changes the fuel system.

By teaching the body to burn fat instead of carbohydrate as its primary energy source it creates a steadier, longer-lasting supply – one that can support long conditioning sessions, and even recovery, without the highs and lows of sugar and carb crashes.

The goal is not to replace one system completely, but to improve how the body manages energy across different demands.

Unlike carbohydrates, which provide quick but limited fuel, burning fat can provides a more stable and sustained energy supply. This is particularly useful for longer training sessions, steady output, and overall energy consistency.

Keto doesn't give you "more energy" – it gives you more usable control over where that energy comes from.

## 3.6 FUEL COMPARISON

At this stage, the key point is simple: Different fuel sources support different types of performance.

Carbohydrates are more useful for short, explosive actions. Fats support longer, more sustained effort.

Boxing requires both.

A fighter needs to be able to produce fast, high-intensity output – but also maintain performance across rounds without fading.

This is why balance matters. Relying too heavily on fast energy can lead to early fatigue if it is not managed properly. Relying only on slower energy can limit sharpness and explosiveness when intensity increases.

The goal is not to choose one fuel system and ignore the other.

It is to understand how they work together and apply them based on the demands of training and competition.

This is where structured nutrition becomes important.

Not guessing. Not reacting. But fuelling with intention.

*Energy Comparison*

| FUEL SOURCE | STORED ENERGY (approx.) | DURATION OF ENERGY | PERFORMANCE EFFECT |
|---|---|---|---|
| Glycogen (Carbs) | 2,000 kcal | 1–2 hours | Fast but limited; leads to crashes |
| Fat Stores | 40,000–80,000 kcal | Many hours | Steady and sustainable energy |

***Coach's Insight:*** *Carbs are like matches – they burn fast. Fat is like coal – steady, strong, and long-lasting.*

**SUMMARY:** ***Fuel, balance, and performance***

Performance depends on how well fuel is managed. Fats support steady energy. Protein supports recovery and strength. Carbohydrates support high-intensity output.

Each has a role, and problems usually come from imbalance – not from the nutrients themselves. When fuel is managed properly, energy becomes more consistent and weight is easier to control. And weight can be lost without starving the body of the energy that it needs.

The next step is applying this knowledge in practice – using structure, timing, and adjustments that match the demands of training.

# ROUND 4

# UNDERSTANDING KETOSIS

## *Fat-Burning State*

Ketosis is the natural metabolic state where your body shifts from burning carbohydrates (glucose) to burning fat (ketones).

The ketogenic diet – often called *keto* – works by pushing the body into a state of ketosis, so that it draws its energy by breaking down fat into ketones, instead of carbohydrate into glucose. Ketogenic diet is one of the most discussed and misunderstood topics in modern nutrition. In some circles, it's promoted as a weight-loss miracle. In others, it's dismissed as a dangerous trend.

But the truth, as always, is more balanced: keto isn't magic, and it isn't madness – it's a method.

That's the focus of this chapter: How keto changes the body's engine and how that affects performance.

Like any tool, its success depends on how and when it's used. When applied with structure, awareness, and proper guidance, the ketogenic diet can help boxers reduce body fat gradually, stabilise energy levels, and improve self-regulation around food – all without starving, dehydrating, or losing power.

That's why this chapter exists. Not to sell keto, but to explain it – clearly, simply, and through the lens of boxing performance. What matters is not hype – it's understanding what's actually happening inside your body, and how it affects your performance.

Keto isn't about eating less – it's about fuelling differently. It changes the body's primary energy source from carbohydrates to fat, offering a steady supply of fuel for training and recovery. For some athletes, that shift can feel freeing.

For others, it may feel restrictive or uncomfortable – especially without the right support.

This chapter doesn't just define keto.

It breaks down why it works, what the diet looks like in practice, and how it can be used as one safe alternative to rushed weight-cutting methods. In boxing, control beats chaos. The more a fighter understands how their body creates, stores, and uses energy, the less they'll rely on panic when it matters most.

## 4.1 WHAT KETO REALLY MEANS

Keto means reprogramming the body's fuel system.

What often fails the boxer is not conditioning, but fuel availability. "Running out of gas" is the moment when the standard carbohydrate fuel runs out.

The ketogenic diet changes that equation. Cutting carbohydrate intake – usually to around 50 grams per day or less – triggers the body begins to fire up its alternative fuel system, shifting from relying on glucose to using fat as its primary fuel. When this system comes into play, the liver breaks down fats into molecules called **ketone bodies**, which are then used by both the muscles and the brain as a steady source of energy.

This natural metabolic shift is known as **ketosis**.

In ketosis, the body becomes more efficient at burning fat – not just from food, but also from stored body fat. Adapting to this alternative fuel source also triggers other effects within the body. Brain cells can use ketones more efficiently than glucose. There is an anti-inflammatory effect that protects all organs including the brain, and a boost to chemicals which help to repair brain cells and build neural networks. That's why some athletes feel more stable energy, less hunger, and sharper focus once fully adapted.

The goal isn't to "starve the body." It's to teach the body a new fuel system – one that can be useful for controlled weight loss, longer training sessions, or building a calm and steady relationship with food.

*Keto doesn't mean eating less.*

A common mistake of low carb-diets is to cut carbohydrate without eating enough fat. This leaves the body with too little fuel overall – leading to low energy, poor recovery, and frustration. If carbs go down, fat intake must go up to replace that energy. Otherwise, performance will drop.

*The goal is not to eat fat for the sake of it.*

The goal is to use fat as a consistent, reliable fuel source that supports training, recovery, and weight control. Because in boxing, energy that lasts is far more valuable than energy that spikes – and disappears. Keto means eating differently – with fat as the star fuel, protein for repair, and carbs kept low and strategic. It's not complicated. But it does require structure, patience, and an understanding of how your body responds.

It's about changing the balance.

*Typical Balance of Nutrients in a Keto Diet Compared to a Standard Diet*

| NUTRIENT | PERCENTAGE OF TOTAL CALORIES | FUNCTION |
|---|---|---|
| Fats | 70–75%<br>*(20-30% in standard diet)* | Primary fuel source<br>*(Secondary in standard diet)* |
| Protein | 20–25%<br>*(Similar to standard diet)* | Muscle repair and recovery |
| Carbohydrates | 5% (approx. 30–50 g/day)<br>*(45-65% in a standard diet)* | Limited and strategic energy source<br>*(Primary source in standard diet)* |

*Values are general guidelines and may vary depending on the individual, training demands, and adaptation level.*

This structure doesn't starve the athlete – it **reprograms metabolism** so the body becomes efficient at burning the fuel it carries the most of: **fat**.

Once adapted to a ketogenic diet, many fighters report more stable energy, fewer cravings, and a clearer hunger signal – not constant thoughts about the next meal. The process of adaptation takes time, however, and this is often a difficult period. The hurdles confronted during the transition to a ketogenic diet is covered in Round 5.

## 4.2 THE BODY'S ENERGY SYSTEMS

To understand how nutrition affects boxing performance, you need to understand how the body actually produces and uses energy.

The body does not switch between energy systems.

All systems are always working together – the difference is how much each one contributes depending on the intensity and duration of the work.

In boxing, this matters.

For short, explosive actions – fast combinations, sharp reactions, sudden bursts – the body relies heavily on glycogen (stored carbohydrates). This system provides fast, powerful energy, but it runs out quickly.

That's why a boxer can feel sharp early in a round – then suddenly flat if that energy isn't supported.

For longer efforts – movement and repeated rounds – the body relies more on fat as a fuel source. This system produces energy more slowly, but it lasts much longer and helps maintain consistency over time.

Both systems are always active. The key is not choosing one – it's understanding how they work together.

A boxer who relies only on fast energy may start strong but struggle to maintain output. A boxer who only focuses on steady energy may lack sharpness and explosiveness when it matters.

High-level performance requires both:

- ✓ Fast energy for explosive exchanges
- ✓ Stable energy for sustained output and control

This is where nutrition becomes important.

A carbohydrate-heavy approach supports high-intensity output but may lead to energy drops if not managed properly.

A fat-adapted approach can improve energy stability, but explosive actions still depend on glycogen. Keto does not replace the need for fast energy. It changes how the body manages and uses fuel.

Even in a fat-adapted athlete, high-intensity actions – combinations, counters, bursts – still rely on glycogen. The goal is not to replace one system with another.

The goal is to build a system that allows you to perform across all demands of boxing.

Because in the ring, it's not about how fast you start.

It's about how well you can maintain your level – and still produce when it matters most.

> ***Coach's Insight:*** *You don't win fights by choosing one energy system. You win by being able to use the right energy at the right time.*

## 4.3 BENEFITS OBSERVED

Once the adaptation phase is complete, many athletes report noticeable changes in both training and recovery.

These are not overnight transformations – they're the result of consistent eating, smart hydration, and listening to how the body responds during each stage of the camp. Common benefits include:

- ✓ **More stable energy throughout the day**. No sugar highs, no post-meal crashes – especially during double sessions.

- ✓ **Sharper focus and calmer mindset**. Ketones provide a steady fuel source for the brain, often improving concentration.
- ✓ **Reduced hunger and better self-control around food**. Higher-fat meals naturally increase satiety (the feeling of fullness) which reduces cravings and emotional eating.
- ✓ **Better fat loss while protecting muscle**. With protein intake maintained, strength and power stay intact while body composition gradually improves.
- ✓ **Less joint stiffness and inflammation.** Some athletes notice improved recovery and reduced soreness – especially during high-volume training blocks.

These benefits aren't guaranteed – they depend on proper planning, hydration, and monitoring. But when the process is respected, the results can create a healthier and more performance-led approach, with general benefits as well as more effective weight control.

---

***Coach's Insight:*** *Stable energy wins fights. Not big spikes – consistency over rounds.*

---

## 4.4 COMMON MYTHS ABOUT KETO

Most confusion around keto in boxing comes from applying it too rigidly or at the wrong time. What works in general fitness doesn't always transfer directly to high-intensity sport. Boxing demands flexibility.

Keto is often marketed as a quick fix, and a lot of misinformation comes with it.

Let's clear a few things up.

*Myths vs Reality*

| MYTH | REALITY |
| --- | --- |
| "Keto is just eating bacon and fats" | It's about quality fats – fish, olive oil, nuts, avocado. Quality of intake matters far more than just eating high fat. |
| "You don't need carbs at all." | Some carbs can be used strategically, especially around high-intensity training.<br>Cutting carbs completely is likely to lead to nutrient deficiencies and potential health risks. |
| "Keto kills performance." | Once properly adapted, many athletes experience stable energy and improved endurance. |
| "It's unsafe." | Used long-term and exclusively, or with poor quality foods, there are potential health risks to a keto diet. When applied correctly, it can be used safely for significant periods and for many people will have significant health benefits. |
| "It works for everyone." | No approach works for everyone. Some perform better on keto, others on balanced carbs. Individual response is key. |

The reality is simple – context matters.

Keto is just one tool. Used properly, it can work. Used blindly, it can backfire. Like anything in boxing – success comes down to **understanding, consistency, and applying it at the right time for the right athlete.**

> ***Coach's Insight:*** *Most people judge keto without ever doing it properly. Poor execution leads to poor results.*

## 4.5 LEARNING FROM REAL EXPERIENCE

In over 35 years of training and coaching, I've seen how much a boxer's energy and mindset can change simply by understanding how the body works.

When food stops being treated as the enemy and starts being respected as fuel, everything shifts – not just physically, but mentally. Fighters who once panicked in fight week begin to stay in control. Instead of guessing, they track what they eat and drink. Instead of feeling drained and desperate, they stay focused and prepared.

When they understand how to use fats and protein properly, energy becomes more stable. The constant thinking about food fades. Attention shifts where it should be – onto performance. That's the real value of this approach. It's not just about losing weight. It's about building awareness.

When nutrition becomes a tool instead of a fear, the boxer becomes:

- ✓ More consistent in training
- ✓ Less emotional about food
- ✓ More confident stepping on the scales
- ✓ More focused on fight night

That's not theory – that's what structure creates.

---

***Coach's Insight:*** *Keto is not a diet to survive; it's a method to understand. Once you learn how your body reacts to food, you control your performance instead of chasing it.*

---

**SUMMARY:** ***Understanding the alternative***

Ketosis changes how the body produces energy, shifting the main fuel source from carbohydrates to fats.

When applied properly, this can support more stable energy, improved weight control, and better consistency during training.

However, it is not a one-size-fits-all approach. Some boxers benefit from it, while others perform better with different strategies.

The key is understanding how your body responds and applying the method in a way that supports performance – not limits it.

# ROUND 5

# TRANSITION AND ADAPTATION

## *A Journey Not a Jump*

The aim of the keto diet is to adjust how body is fuelled and produces energy. That's adaptation. Getting there doesn't happen all at once. The shift from carbohydrate-based energy to fat-based energy is a physiological process that takes time. It involves a period of transition that is often challenging.

This early phase of keto is where most mistakes happen.

Not because the system fails – but because it is misunderstood.

This phase is not where the system breaks. It is where it begins to work.

This round focuses on what this journey actually feels like, what is happening in the body, and how to manage it without losing control.

Because when you understand the transition, it won't make you panic.

---

***Coach's Insight:*** *The first stage of keto isn't about toughness – it's about teaching your body a new fuel system. Give it time to adapt.*

---

## 5.1 TRANSITION (WEEK-BY-WEEK)

Moving into keto should not be rushed. A structured transition allows the body to adjust while maintaining control over training and performance.

This is a practical framework for managing that transition.

*Week-by-Week Keto Transition Plan*

| WEEK | FOCUS | TRAINING EMPHASIS | NOTES |
|---|---|---|---|
| 1 | Reduce carbs to 100-120 g/day | Technical drills and moderate intensity | Increase hydration; note early changes |
| 2 | Reduce carbs to 60-80 g/day | Aerobic conditioning & skills work | Mild fatigue normal; keep session steady |
| 3-4 | 30-50 g/day (keto range) | Controlled sparring and intervals | Energy steadier – body adapting |
| 5+ | Maintain adapted state | 5% (approx. 30–50 g/day) | Monitor sleep, focus, recovery |

The timescales in this plan should be treated as a guide, not a rule. Transition is unlikely to take less time than indicated here, but can take longer depending on:

- Consistency in nutrition
- Training intensity
- Hydration and recovery

- Individual response

Some athletes adapt quickly. Others take more time.

The key is not speed.

The key is consistency.

## WEEK 1 – REDUCE AND ADJUST

The focus here is on reducing carbohydrate intake gradually, not eliminating everything at once.

At the same time:

- Increase fat intake to support energy
- Maintain consistent protein intake
- Prioritise hydration and electrolyte balance

Training should be adjusted slightly:

- Lower overall intensity if needed
- Focus on technical work and controlled sessions

The goal is not peak performance – it's a smooth start.

*What is happening?*

With the reduction in carbohydrate, glycogen stores are depleted and cannot be wholly replaced. The body is therefore very short of its normal fuel.

However it takes up to a week before ketosis kicks in to provide an alternative fuel. As a result, the body struggles to find energy, and may briefly start burning protein to create glucose.

At the same time, hydration levels shift.

Glycogen stores include a lot of water, and as glycogen stores decrease, this water is shed, which will result in a rapid once-off weight loss.

Electrolytes (the minerals that regulate nerve and muscle function) are affected. This can influence how the body feels in training and contributes to fatigue if not managed properly.

This first week may be difficult. As described below many people experience "keto flu" at this time, with headaches, fatigue, and irritability, along with rapid water loss, increased thirst and a craving for carbs,.

This is temporary.

---

***Coach's Insight:*** *The first week is not the result. It's the adjustment. Judge progress over weeks – not days.*

---

WEEK 2 – STABILISE AND OBSERVE

By now, the body is beginning to shift.

Focus on:

- Consistency in nutrition

- Stable daily structure
- Maintaining recovery habits

Training can begin to increase slightly:

- Reintroduce moderate intensity
- Keep volume controlled

The key here is patience. Avoid making big changes too quickly.

*What is happening?*

During this period, the body is caught between two systems.

It is still expecting carbohydrates and attuned to getting energy from glycogen, so the loss of carbs may still be producing uncomfortable symptoms.

Ketosis is kicking in and the liver is starting to convert fat into ketone for energy. However, the production of ketones may be limited and fluctuating. The new fuel is also unfamiliar, and until the body has adapted to it, it cannot use ketones efficiently.

As a result, performance may feel inconsistent. This is not a lack of fitness. It is a shift in fuel use. Some sessions feel normal. Others feel flat. Output may drop earlier than expected, and reactions may feel slightly slower. Energy may fluctuate. Output may not match expectations. This is where many boxers make the wrong decision. They feel a drop in performance, assume the system is failing, and stop too early.

This is not failure. It is the transition.

---

***Coach's Insight:*** *Most boxers rush the first two weeks. Then they say it doesn't work. Give the body time to adjust, keep the structure, and stay consistent. That's where the real results come from.*

---

## WEEK 3 – BUILD AND REINFORCE

The body is becoming more efficient at using fat for fuel.

Now you can:

- Increase training intensity gradually
- Add more demanding sessions
- Maintain structure in nutrition

*What is happening?*

The body is learning to use a different fuel system.

Production of ketones from fat is becoming more consistent and efficient. Hunger and craving for carbohydrates may be starting to fade.

At the same time, the body is beginning to adapt to the new fuel. There is an increase in the structures within body and brain cells (mitochondria) which convert fuel sources to energy. This improves the body's metabolism and its ability to use ketones efficiently.

As this process develops, energy delivery starts to become more stable and less dependent on carbohydrate intake. These gains are incomplete, so their benefits may not yet be felt and there will still be "off days"

***Coach's Insight:*** *Feeling off doesn't mean it's wrong. It means something is changing. The mistake is quitting before it settles.*

WEEK 4 – RETURN TO PERFORMANCE

At this stage, the goal is to return to normal training demands.

You should be able to:

- Handle higher intensity work
- Maintain consistent output
- Recover effectively between sessions

From here, adjustments become individual. Some boxers may need small changes depending on how they respond.

The transition phase is not about perfection. It's about control.

A structured approach keeps everything moving in the right direction.

*What is happening?*

The body is becoming efficient at burning fat. Ketone levels in the blood may drop compared to early keto stages because the body uses them more efficiently. This further reduces some of the negative experiences of the earlier weeks.

Hunger vanishes due to improved satiety signalling, and physical stamina often stabilizes or improves.

Other beneficial effects of ketosis are also beginning to take effect. The increase in mitochondria improves muscle endurance, and overall metabolism becomes more efficient.

As adaptation is established, the body is able to produce energy in a more stable and sustainable way, supporting longer sessions and improved control over body weight.

## 5.2 WHAT HAPPENS DURING THE TRANSITION

During this phase, training should be managed carefully. This is not the time to push maximum intensity. Focus on technical work, movement, and controlled conditioning while the body adapts.

This is why the transition phase is often misunderstood.

The issue is not the approach itself, but how the body is responding to the change. With proper structure, hydration, and patience, this phase stabilises.

> ***Coach's Insight:*** *Most early problems aren't the diet. They're the transition. Understand what's changing, and you stop reacting to it.*

### 5.3 COMMON SYMPTOMS (KETO FLU)

Some boxers experience what is commonly referred to as the "keto flu."

This is not an illness. It is a temporary response to changes in fuel use and hydration.

Common symptoms may include:

- Low energy
- Headaches
- Reduced training output
- Mild dizziness
- Increased fatigue

These symptoms are usually short-term and often linked to:

- Low electrolyte intake

- Dehydration
- Sudden carbohydrate reduction

When managed properly, they pass. The key is not to panic and overcorrect.

Small adjustments – especially in hydration and electrolytes – usually resolve the issue.

## 5.4 ADAPTATION

Adaptation is achieved as the body becomes more efficient at using fat and ketones as a primary fuel source.

Over time, the body improves its ability to produce and use ketones effectively. This often begins around weeks three and four of the transition,

When the process is managed properly, energy becomes more stable, training becomes more predictable, and performance begins to normalise.

---

***Coach's Insight:*** *Your body doesn't switch systems overnight. It learns. Give it time to adjust, not pressure to perform immediately.*

---

**SUMMARY:** ***Understanding transition and adaptation***

This is the phase where most doubt appears. Performance may feel inconsistent. Energy may fluctuate. Training may feel harder than expected.

This is not failure. It is part of the process.

When managed properly, the body adjusts, energy stabilises, and performance becomes more consistent again.

The key is not to avoid the phase – but to stay controlled and disciplined while moving through it.

# ROUND 6

# APPLYING KETO IN BOXING

## *From Theory to Practice*

Understanding keto is one thing. Applying it properly is something else. This is where most boxers get it wrong. They take an idea, follow it blindly, and expect it to work – without considering timing, training demands, or how their body responds. That's not strategy. That's guesswork.

In boxing, everything has to fit the bigger picture. Training, recovery, weight management, and performance are all connected. Nutrition is not separate – it has to support the system.

This round is about turning knowledge into action. When keto makes sense. How to plan it. How to transition without losing performance. And how to adjust based on what's actually happening – not what you expected to happen. Because the goal is not to follow a diet. The goal is to make decisions that improve performance. And that requires structure, awareness, and control.

*Important Note:*

> This chapter offers general guidance, not individual medical advice. Before starting or adapting any ketogenic or low-carbohydrate plan, every boxer should consult a qualified dietitian, sports nutritionist, or other relevant healthcare professional. This is particularly

important for women boxers, because of the potential impact of a keto diet on female hormones, and for any boxer who has a medical condition or is taking medication.

## 6.1 WHEN KETO MAKES SENSE

Keto is not for everyone. And it's not something a boxer should follow just because it's popular, trending, or worked for someone else. It has to make sense for the individual. The key is understanding **when it helps performance – and when it doesn't.** Keto tends to work best for boxers who:

- Struggle with constant weight fluctuations
- Find themselves in repeated cut-and-rebound cycles
- Feel energy crashes during the day
- Over-rely on sugar or quick carbohydrates
- Need better appetite control and consistency

In these cases, keto can bring structure, stability, and better long-term control. It can also be useful during:

- Off-season phases
- Lower-intensity training periods
- Base conditioning blocks
- Longer-term body composition work

Here, the goal is not just performance in a single session – but building a more efficient and controlled system over time. However, keto may not be the best approach when:

- Training is highly explosive and glycolytic

- Sessions rely heavily on repeated high intensity output
- The boxer is already lean and performing well
- There is limited time before competition
- The athlete responds poorly to low carbohydrate intake, even after the initial transition phase

In these situations, a more mixed or targeted approach may be more effective. The most important point is this: there is no single diet that works for every boxer. The goal is not to follow keto. The goal is to **understand your body – and use the right approach at the right time.**

A good boxer doesn't just train hard. They learn how to manage their system. And nutrition is part of that system – not separate from it.

***Coach's Insight:*** *Most boxers don't need a new diet. They need better timing. Keto isn't good or bad – it's situational. Use it when it fits the phase, not when it's popular.*

## 6.2 PLANNING AND MONITORING

Starting keto without a plan is one of the biggest mistakes a boxer can make. It's not something where you "suck it and see." It needs structure from the start.

The first step is clarity. You need to know:

- Why you're doing it
- What phase of training you're in
- What outcome you're aiming for (weight loss, weight control, energy stability, body composition)

Without that, there's no direction – just random changes.

Next is setting a clear approach. This includes:

- Reducing carbohydrate intake in a controlled way
- Increasing fats to support energy
- Keeping protein consistent for recovery and muscle maintenance

At the same time, hydration and electrolytes must be managed properly. This is where many boxers struggle early on – not because keto doesn't work, but because they don't support the process correctly.

Monitoring is just as important as planning. You need to pay attention to:

- Energy levels during training
- Performance (especially in high-intensity work)
- Recovery between sessions
- Body weight and how it fluctuates

This isn't about overcomplicating things. It's about staying aware. Adjustments should be small and controlled. Not every bad session means something is wrong. But consistent patterns – low energy, poor recovery, performance drop – need to be addressed. A good plan is not fixed. It evolves based on feedback from the body. That's how you stay in control and avoid unnecessary setbacks.

***Coach's Insight:*** *A plan only works if you pay attention. Most boxers don't monitor anything – they just hope it works. Track what matters, make small adjustments, and stay consistent. That's how progress actually happens.*

## 6.3 PERIODISATION

Even once adaptation is achieved, keto is not an unchanging "steady state". It is not something that needs to be followed the same way all year round. In boxing, training changes – and nutrition must change with it. This is where periodisation becomes essential. Different phases of training place different demands on the body. What supports performance in one phase may not be optimal in another. There is no single approach that fits every stage of preparation.

*Off-Season / Base Phase*

This is where keto can work very well. The focus here is:

- Building aerobic capacity
- Improving body composition
- Creating stable energy systems

Lower carbohydrate intake can help:

- Improve fat utilisation
- Avoid unnecessary weight gain

- Maintain consistency without constant fluctuations

This is where the foundation is built.

*Pre-Camp / Early Camp*

As training intensity begins to increase, adjustments may be needed. Some boxers may stay fully keto. Others may introduce small, targeted carbohydrates around training.

The goal is to support performance without losing control.

*Fight Camp / High-Intensity Phase*

This is where demands are highest. Training becomes:

- Faster
- More explosive
- More dependent on fast carbohydrate energy system (more glycolytic)

At this stage, a strict keto approach may not suit every boxer. Options include:

- Targeted carbohydrate use around sessions
- A more flexible, mixed approach

The key is performance. Not sticking rigidly to one method.

*Fight Week / Weight Management*

This phase is highly individual. Keto may help with:

- Appetite control

- Water balance
- Reducing last-minute fluctuations

But it must be managed carefully. No drastic changes. No experiments. Only what has already been tested. This is addressed in more detail in Round 10.

**Key Principle:**

Nutrition should match the phase of training. Not the other way around.

Periodisation allows a boxer to stay in control of weight, maintain energy and support performance when it matters most. Instead of forcing one approach all year round, you adjust based on demand. That's how you train intelligently.

*Keto Periodisation for Boxing*

| PHASE | GOAL | BEST APPROACH |
|---|---|---|
| Off-Season | Reset habits, improve metabolic control | Moderate-carb or cyclical keto |
| Early Camp | Fat adaptation, aerobic conditioning | Full keto for 4-6 weeks |
| Mid Camp | Stabilise and sharpen | Targeted keto with timed carbs |
| Fight Week | Fine-tune fuel and hydration | Limited and strategic energy source |

***Coach's Insight:*** *The mistake is trying to use one system all year. Smart boxers adapt their nutrition. Match the method to the moment – that's where performance improves.*

## 6.4 RED FLAGS

Keto is a tool. But like any tool, it only works when it's used correctly. Ignoring warning signs and pushing through regardless will only trigger problems. One of the biggest mistakes is assuming that every drop in performance is part of the process. Short-term adjustments are normal. But ongoing issues are not.

*Common Red Flags*

Pay attention if you notice:

- Consistently low energy during training
- Poor recovery between sessions
- Loss of strength or sharpness
- Reduced ability to handle intensity
- Ongoing fatigue that doesn't improve

These are not signs to ignore. They are signals that something needs adjusting. It doesn't always mean keto is wrong. But it may mean:

- The timing is not right
- The training demands are too high for the current approach

- Nutrition is not structured properly (calories, fats, electrolytes)
- The boxer is not adapting well to low carbohydrate intake

*When to Adjust*

Adjustments should be controlled and specific. This might include:

- ✓ Slightly increasing carbohydrate intake
- ✓ Adjusting training intensity or volume
- ✓ Improving hydration and electrolyte balance
- ✓ Reviewing overall calorie intake

The first goal is not to abandon the plan immediately. It's to refine it.

*When to Stop*

In some cases, keto may simply not be the right fit. If performance continues to drop despite proper structure and adjustments, a different approach may be more effective. There is no benefit in forcing something that clearly isn't working.

Key principle:

- ✓ Listen to the body
- ✓ But interpret it correctly
- ✓ Not every bad session matters
- ✓ But consistent patterns do

The best decisions are based on observation, not assumption. That's how you avoid unnecessary setbacks and stay on track.

*How to Read Your Body*

| AREA | HEALTHY SIGNS | RED FLAGS / CONCERNS |
|---|---|---|
| Energy | Consistent through session | Sudden fatigue, dizziness, loss of strength |
| Mood | Focused, calm | Irritable, withdrawn, anxious |
| Hydration | Clear urine, good recovery | Dark urine, headaches, cramping |
| Weight trend | Gradual 0.5-1kg per week | Rapid drops, 1.5kg or more per week |
| Performance | Stable or improving | Sharp decline, slow reactions |

***Coach's Insight:*** *Pushing through everything is not discipline. It's poor judgement. If something isn't working, adjust it. That's how you stay in control and keep performance moving forward.*

## 6.5 WORKING AS A TEAM

Nutrition is not just the boxer's responsibility. It is part of the wider system. The coach, the boxer, and the support team all play a role in making it work. That team may include parents or guardians, a dietitian or nutritionist, a strength and conditioning coach, and anyone involved in the athlete's preparation.

Each role brings something different – but they all influence how the boxer trains, fuels, and recovers. A boxer may follow the plan, but if the coach is unaware of the approach, training may not match the demands. At the same time, a coach may push intensity without understanding how the boxer is fuelling.

This is where problems begin. Communication is what keeps the system working. Everyone involved should understand:

- the goal of the approach
- the current phase of training
- any adjustments being made
- how the boxer is responding

This doesn't need to be complicated – but it needs to be clear. The coach should:

- adjust training when needed
- monitor performance and fatigue
- keep sessions aligned with the boxer's current state

The boxer should:

- follow the plan consistently
- be honest about how they feel
- report any issues early

The wider team should:

- support the agreed approach
- avoid conflicting advice
- help maintain consistency around the boxer

When everyone works together, decisions become clearer. Small problems are addressed early, and the process stays controlled.

Key Principle: Performance is not built in isolation. It is built through coordination. The stronger the communication, the smoother the process – and the better the outcome.

---

***Coach's Insight:*** *Most problems don't come from the plan. They come from poor communication. When the boxer and coach are not aligned, performance suffers. Stay connected, stay clear – that's how you keep everything working.*

---

**SUMMARY:** ***Keto is not enough***

Applying it correctly is what makes the difference. In this round, you've seen that success doesn't come from following a diet blindly. It comes from knowing:

- When it makes sense
- How to plan it properly
- When to adjust
- And how to work as a team

Keto is not a fixed system. It's a tool that needs to match the demands of training, the phase of preparation, and how the boxer responds.

The biggest mistake is trying to force it.

The right approach is to guide it. Small adjustments, clear structure, and consistent monitoring are what keep performance moving in the right direction.

When done properly, keto can improve control, stability, and long-term consistency. But only if it's applied with awareness. Because the goal is not to follow a method. The goal is to improve performance. And that always comes down to making the right decisions at the right time.

# ROUND 7

# HYDRATION AND ELECTROLYTES

## *Balancing Fluids for Performance and Control*

Most fighters think hydration just means drinking more water. That's not enough. Hydration is not just about how much you drink – it's about how well your body can **use that fluid**.

When you move into a ketogenic approach, things change. In the first phase, as you adjust to lower carbs, you lose the water that carbohydrates retain in the body. With this, you lose some minerals, particularly sodium. The lower level of water retention will be a consistent feature as long as you maintain the keto approach, but if you don't replace the minerals that you may lose with that water, performance drops fast. Low energy. Cramping. Poor recovery. Flat sessions. Many fighters blame the diet. In reality, they're just **under-mineralised and possibly under-hydrated**. This is where electrolytes come in. Sodium, potassium, and magnesium are not optional – they are essential for:

- muscle function
- nerve signalling
- energy levels
- overall performance

Get this wrong, and everything feels harder than it should. Get it right, and training becomes more stable, more consistent, and more controlled. In this round, you'll learn:

- why hydration works differently on keto
- how dehydration affects performance
- how to manage electrolytes properly
- how to apply hydration strategies in training and fight week

This is one of the most overlooked areas in boxing – and one of the easiest to fix.

## 7.1 WHY HYDRATION MATTERS

Hydration is one of the simplest things in boxing – and one of the most overlooked. Every system in the body depends on it. Your blood volume, temperature control, muscle function, and energy production all rely on proper fluid balance. When hydration drops, performance follows quickly. Even a small level of dehydration can lead to:

- reduced endurance
- slower reactions
- increased fatigue
- higher heart rate during training

In boxing, that means less output, slower combinations, and poorer decision-making.

On a ketogenic approach, your baseline hydration level is lower, and hydration becomes even more important, because there is less leeway for losing fluid. Keto changes how fluid is held and used inside the body. As a result, relying on thirst alone is not enough. By the time you feel thirsty, performance may already be affected. This is why hydration needs to be more controlled and consistent. It's not just about drinking more water – it's about maintaining the right balance of fluids and minerals so the body can function properly.

When the balance is right, energy remains stable, muscles contract efficiently, and recovery is supported. When it's not, fatigue builds faster, output drops, and performance becomes harder to maintain.

Hydration is not just a background factor. It directly affects how well you can train, recover, and perform.

> ***Coach's Insight:*** *If you feel flat, heavy, or tired early in a session, don't assume it's your fitness. Most of the time, it's poor hydration. Fix that first before you question everything else.*

## 7.2 DEHYDRATION EFFECTS

On keto, you should never restrict your fluid intake. You don't need to worry that drinking water will put back the water-weight that you lost when you started keto – the body will only absorb the water that it needs, and the rest will be discarded.

Dehydration, on the other hand, doesn't just make you feel thirsty – it affects how your body performs at every level.

When fluid levels drop, blood volume decreases. This reduces aerobic efficiency and increases perceived effort, even at lower intensities. As a result, fatigue comes earlier, and endurance drops. Muscle function is affected as well. Every contraction depends on proper fluid and electrolyte balance. When hydration is low, muscles don't contract as efficiently. Power drops, reactions slow down, coordination suffers, and the risk of cramping increases.

The brain is just as affected. Even mild dehydration – around 2% of body weight – has been shown to reduce concentration and reaction time. In boxing, that's not small. That's timing, awareness and decision-making – the things that decide rounds.

Temperature regulation is another key factor. The body relies on fluid to control heat through sweating. When you're dehydrated, this system becomes less effective. Core temperature rises faster, fatigue increases, and training intensity becomes harder to sustain.

On a ketogenic approach, because you are carrying much less water, dehydration effects can show up more quickly. Additionally, until you are fully adapted, keto can result in the body losing more sodium through urine, which further disrupts fluid balance. This is why dehydration on keto is often misunderstood. It's not just about water – it's about fluid *and* minerals.

Poor hydration may not always leave you feeling thirsty, but performance will already be affected:

- energy drops earlier
- output becomes inconsistent
- recovery slows down

That's why dehydration is not something to react to. It's something to prevent. This is where electrolytes become critical – and why hydration is more than just water. We'll break that down next.

---

***Coach's Insight:*** *If your performance drops halfway through a session, look at your hydration before anything else. You can't out-train dehydration.*

---

## 7.3 ELECTROLYTES

Hydration is not just about water. Without electrolytes, water alone doesn't work properly in the body. You can drink more and still feel flat if the balance isn't right. Electrolytes are minerals that control how fluid moves in and out of your cells. They also allow your muscles to contract and your nerves to send signals. Without them, fluid balance breaks down and the system cannot function efficiently.

The main ones to focus on are **sodium**, **potassium**, and **magnesium**. These are not optional – they are essential for performance. When electrolyte levels are balanced, everything works the way it should. Muscles contract properly, nerves fire efficiently, and energy systems run smoothly. You feel more stable, more responsive, and more in control during training.

But when those levels drop, everything becomes harder – even if you're drinking enough water. This is where many fighters go wrong. They increase their water intake but don't replace electrolytes. That creates an imbalance. The body has fluid, but it can't use it properly. That's when problems start to show. Energy drops, headaches appear, you feel dizzy or flat, muscles tighten or cramp, and sessions don't feel sharp. It's not always obvious at first, but over time it affects performance more and more.

This is an issue for athletes whatever their diet, but on a ketogenic approach, this becomes even more important. Keto results in lower insulin levels and this causes the body to lose more sodium through urine. And when sodium drops, other electrolytes tend to follow. This is one of the main reasons behind what people call the "keto flu." It's not just the diet. It's the loss of minerals. When electrolytes are managed properly, the difference is clear. Energy improves, hydration actually works, and performance becomes more stable. Sessions feel more consistent instead of unpredictable.

---

***Coach's Insight:*** *If you're drinking more water but still feel flat, don't assume you need to push harder. You're not lacking effort. You're lacking electrolytes.*

---

## 7.4 DAILY GUIDELINES

Hydration needs to be consistent. It's not something you fix during training – it starts before the session and continues throughout the day.

A simple approach works best. Start with regular water intake spread across the day rather than large amounts at once. This helps maintain stable fluid levels instead of constant ups and downs.

But don't just focus on water. Drinking large amounts without replacing electrolytes can make things worse, not better. Alongside water, electrolytes need to be included daily – not just when you feel tired. A practical baseline:

- add a little salt to meals regularly
- consider a pinch of salt in water, especially in the morning
- regularly eat foods rich in potassium and magnesium, such as leafy greens, nuts, seeds, and salmon
- increase intake on harder training days

Unless advised otherwise by a health professional, it is better to raise electrolytes through careful choice of natural foods rather than through supplements such as "sports drinks" or pills. You can get all the electrolytes you need from natural foods, but (with the exception of salt, which it is easy to take to excess) you won't get too many electrolytes that way. Adding too many electrolytes from artificial supplements is easy, however. This can cause problems, including high blood pressure and heart irregularities. To compound the risks, the signs of excess electrolytes can seem similar to those caused by insufficient electrolytes, including fatigue and confusion. If this mistakenly leads to increasing electrolyte consumption, the problems will then spiral.

You don't need complicated formulas. What matters is consistency and a healthy intake of appropriate foods.

Signs your hydration is on track:

- stable energy levels
- no early fatigue in sessions
- minimal cramping
- steady focus

Signs it's not:

- feeling flat or heavy
- headaches
- sudden drops in performance
- needing excessive water during training

On a ketogenic approach, daily hydration needs attention. To maintain the right balance, drink plenty, eat natural foods, consistently, every day. When that balance is right, energy stays stable, training feels controlled, and performance holds up. When it's not, everything starts to slip – often without you realising why.

***Coach's Insight:*** *Don't wait until you feel dehydrated. By then, performance is already dropping. Stay ahead of it.*

## 7.5 TRAINING HYDRATION

Hydration is not about reacting – it's about preparation. If you start a session already dehydrated, you spend the whole time trying to catch up. Performance will suffer, no matter how hard you push. The goal is simple: arrive hydrated, maintain it during the session, and restore it afterwards.

**Before training:** Start the session properly hydrated. This comes from consistent intake throughout the day, not from trying to fix it just before you begin.

**During training:** Small, regular sips work better than large amounts at once. This helps maintain fluid balance without discomfort.

**After training:** Rehydration is part of recovery. Replacing both fluids and electrolytes supports muscle function and reduces fatigue going into the next session.

**Fight week:** Managing hydration during fight week requires particular care, although the principles remain the same. The challenges of fight week are covered in Round 10.

***Coach's Insight:*** *If your performance is inconsistent from session to session, check your hydration first.*

## 7.6 COMMON MISTAKES

From all the above, the mistakes to avoid should be clear:

- Don't just focus on water. Remember the electrolytes. Something as simple as adding a small pinch of salt (such as sea salt or Himalayan salt) to water can help restore balance more effectively than water alone.
- Don't react too late. By the point you feel tired, cramped, or lightheaded, your performance has already dropped.
- Don't chop and change your daily regime. Hydrating well one day and neglecting it the next leads to unstable performance.
- Don't overcomplicate things. Hydration needs attention but it is not complicated and does not require a magic formula: just stick to simple, consistent habits that actually work.

During fight week, mistakes become more extreme. These issues are addressed in Round 10.

***Coach's Insight:*** *Keep it simple. Most fighters don't need a better system – they need to follow a basic one properly every day.*

**SUMMARY:** ***Hydration drives performance***

It's about maintaining the right balance of fluids and electrolytes so the body can function properly. Without that balance, performance drops and on a ketogenic approach, this shows up faster, through fatigue, reduced output, and inconsistent performance. Electrolytes – especially sodium, potassium, and magnesium – are essential.

Keep it simple. Stay consistent. Get the basics right, and performance becomes more stable, more reliable, and easier to maintain.

# ROUND 8

# TRAINING ON KETO

## *Adapting Performance to a New Fuel System*

Understanding how the body uses fuel is one thing. Applying it in training is another. This is where most doubts come in. Can you perform without relying on high carbohydrates? Will power drop? Will conditioning suffer? These questions are common – especially in a sport like boxing, where intensity, speed, and endurance all matter. The reality is more nuanced.

In this round, you'll learn:

- how energy systems apply to boxing performance
- what to expect when training on keto
- how to structure strength and conditioning
- how to use carbohydrates strategically when needed

This is where theory becomes practice. And where the system either works – or fails – depending on how it's applied.

### 8.1 ENERGY AND PERFORMANCE

By this point, you understand how the body produces energy – and how different fuels support different types of work. Now the focus is simple: *how that actually shows up in training*. Because this is where theory meets reality. In boxing, performance is not one thing. It's a combination of:

- Explosive actions (combinations, counters, reactions)
- Sustained effort (movement, pacing, repeated rounds)
- Mental sharpness (timing, decisions under pressure)

Each of these places different demands on the body. And no single fuel system covers all of them perfectly. This is where many boxers get it wrong. They follow an approach – high-carb or keto – and expect it to solve everything. But performance doesn't work like that.

A carbohydrate-heavy approach can support high-intensity output. But if poorly managed, it can lead to energy drops, poor control, and reliance on constant refuelling.

A fat-adapted approach can improve energy stability and consistency. But high-intensity actions still depend on glycogen – that doesn't change.

So the question is not: *"Which system is better?"*

The question is: *"Does your current approach support the demands of your training?"*

This is where awareness becomes important. If you feel:

- Sharp early, but fading quickly → fast energy is there, but not sustained
- Stable, but lacking explosiveness → steady energy is there, but output is limited
- Flat across sessions → overall fuel or recovery is not supporting the work

These are not random issues. They are feedback. Keto does not automatically improve performance. It can improve control, stability, and consistency – but only if it fits the demands of training. In practice, many boxers find that:

- Lower-intensity sessions feel more controlled when fat-adapted
- Longer sessions feel more stable
- But high-intensity work may still require targeted carbohydrate support

That's not a contradiction. That's how the body works. The goal is not to force one system. The goal is to build a system that allows you to:

- Maintain energy across rounds
- Deliver when it matters
- Recover between sessions
- Stay in control of your weight

Because in boxing, performance is not about feeling good at one point. It's about being able to repeat output – under fatigue, under pressure, round after round.

---

***Coach's Insight:*** *Performance is not about choosing a diet. It's about matching your fuel to your work – and adjusting when it doesn't match.*

---

## 8.2 STRENGTH AND CONDITIONING

Strength and conditioning on a ketogenic approach doesn't change what you train – it changes how your body supports that work.

Under normal conditions, high-intensity efforts rely heavily on glycogen. This is stored carbohydrate used for short, explosive actions like sprints, powerful combinations, and maximal lifts. On a lower-carbohydrate approach, glycogen availability is reduced, especially in the early stages. That doesn't mean strength disappears – but it does mean the body has to work differently. Once adapted, the body becomes more efficient at using fat for longer-duration efforts and recovery between bouts of work. This can support sustained output across sessions, but very high-intensity efforts may feel more demanding if not managed properly. From a training perspective, this means structure matters.

Strength work can still be maintained – especially when sessions are controlled and quality-focused. Lower rep ranges, recovery between sets, and good technical execution allow the body to produce force without relying heavily on rapid glycogen use.

Conditioning work may need slight adjustment, particularly during adaptation. Instead of relying only on repeated high-intensity bursts, sessions can include more controlled intervals and aerobic-based work to support the shift in energy systems. As adaptation improves, the body becomes better at switching between fuel sources. This allows for more flexibility – combining steady energy from fat with targeted use of carbohydrates when needed.

The key point is this: the goal is not train less – it's to match training to the system you're using. When training is aligned with how the body is fuelled, performance becomes more stable, recovery improves, and output can be maintained across rounds and sessions.

> ***Coach's Insight:*** *If your strength drops, don't blame the diet straight away. Check your structure first. Most problems come from how you train – not how you eat.*

## 8.3 STRATEGIC CARBOHYDRATE USE

A ketogenic approach does not mean carbohydrates must be completely avoided at all times. It means they are used with purpose. In boxing, there are situations where small, controlled amounts of carbohydrates can be useful – especially around high-intensity work. These may include:

- hard sparring sessions
- intense conditioning work
- competition periods

The reason is simple. High-intensity efforts rely on glycogen – stored carbohydrate in the muscles. When glycogen is low, repeated explosive efforts become harder to maintain. Small, targeted carbohydrate intake can help restore glycogen levels and support these demands without disrupting the overall system. The key is control. Instead of relying on carbohydrates throughout the day, they are used strategically to support specific sessions. This allows you to maintain the benefits of a ketogenic approach while still supporting peak performance when needed. However, this needs to be applied carefully. Uncontrolled intake can disrupt adaptation and lead to unstable energy levels. The goal is not to move in and out of the system randomly, but to use carbohydrates deliberately when they serve a clear purpose.

For example, a boxer may use a small amount of faster-digesting carbohydrates before a hard sparring session, intense conditioning workout, or competition where explosive output is required. Faster–digesting carbohydrates may include foods such as bananas, honey, white rice, rice cakes or small amounts of glucose–based drinks. These can provide energy more quickly and may help support repeated high intensity efforts.

Slower–digesting carbohydrates, such as oats, brown rice, sweet potatoes, quinoa, or wholegrain foods, release energy more gradually and may be more suitable eaten earlier before training sessions or during heaver training periods.

Some fighters may perform well with targeted "fast" carbohydrates 30-60 minutes before training, while others may prefer a "slower" carbohydrates 2-3 hours before the session.

During very demanding or longer sessions, small amounts of carbs and electrolytes may also help support performance and reduce fatigue.

For many fighters, this may not be necessary all the time. Some will perform well without additional carbohydrates, especially once fully adapted. Others may benefit from small, targeted use depending on training intensity and individual response. There is no single rule.

What matters is understanding your body and applying the approach consistently. Strategic use is not about adding more. It's about using the right amount, at the right time, for the right reason.

**Attention:** while some athletes rely heavily on popular energy drinks or isotonic products, many of these are highly processed, high in added sugars, artificial flavourings, colourings, and unnecessary stimulants. Regular use can lead to unstable energy levels, poor nutritional habits, and over-reliance on quick sugar intake rather than proper fuelling strategies.

Whenever possible, more natural carbohydrates sources are better option. Simple homemade drinks such as water mixed with small amounts of honey, fresh lemon, sea salt, or blended fruit can help support hydration and energy levels without relying on highly processed products.

***Coach's Insight:*** *Carbs shouldn't be used by default. Use them when they serve a purpose – not out of habit.*

## 8.4 ADJUSTING TRAINING TO THE SYSTEM

Adjusting training to a ketogenic approach is not about lowering standards – it's about matching the work to how the body is currently fuelled. This means aligning intensity, volume, and recovery with how energy is actually being produced – not how it was produced before. Every training session places a demand on the body. That demand has to be met by the available energy system.

When carbohydrate intake is reduced, the body relies less on rapid glycogen use and more on slower, more stable fuel sources. This doesn't limit performance – but it does change how that performance is best expressed. High-intensity efforts that depend on fast, repeated bursts of energy can feel more demanding, especially if recovery between efforts is too short. This is because glycogen availability is lower, and the body needs more time to regenerate usable energy. This is where small adjustments make a difference.

Managing rest periods becomes more important. Slightly longer recovery between high-intensity efforts allows the body to restore energy more effectively, helping maintain quality across rounds or sets.

Session structure also matters.

- ✓ Instead of stacking multiple high-intensity efforts back-to-back, spacing them out or combining them with lower-intensity work can improve overall output and reduce early fatigue.
- ✓ Training volume and intensity don't need to drop – but they need to be organised with purpose.
- ✓ Quality becomes more important than simply pushing through fatigue.

As adaptation improves, the body becomes more efficient at using available fuel and recovering between efforts. This allows for greater flexibility, including the ability to handle more demanding sessions when required.

The key point is this: performance doesn't just depend on how hard you train – it depends on how well your training matches the system supporting it. When training is structured around how the body produces energy, sessions become more consistent, output is easier to maintain, and fatigue is better managed across the week.

---

***Coach's Insight:*** *If something feels off, don't force it. Adjust, don't fight the system.*

---

*Example Week*

*Fat – Adapted Boxer during weight reduction(keto-based approach with targeted carbohydrate use)*

| DAY | TRAINING FOCUS | NUTRITION FOCUS | PRACTICAL GIDELINES |
|---|---|---|---|
| MON | **Technical**<br>**Strength** | High fat, adequate protein | Standard keto meals, maintain hydration |
| TUE | **Conditioning**<br>**Core** | High fat, adequate protein, hydration and electrolytes | Standard keto meals, (add magnesium, potassium-rich foods: leafy greens, avocado, oily fish). Hydration (water with sea salt, mineral water) |
| WED | **Tactics**<br>**Sparring** | High fat, adequate protein, + 20-40g fast carbs pre-session | Standard keto meals, (plus banana, rice cakes before session), maintain hydration |
| THU | **Mobility**<br>**Tactics** | High fat, adequate protein, maintain hydration | Standard keto meals, maintain hydration |
| FRI | **Technical**<br>**Sparring** | High fat, adequate protein, + 20-40g carbs pre-session | Standard keto meals, (plus pre-session banana, rice cakes), maintain hydration |
| SAT | **Conditioning** | High fat, adequate protein, hydration + electrolytes | Standard keto meals, (add mineral-rich foods: leafy greens, avocado, sardines, mackerel). Hydration (water with sea salt, mineral water) |
| SUN | **Rest** | High fat, adequate protein, maintain hydration | Check weight, make notes, adjust training and fuel for next week |

**SUMMARY:** ***Performance is built, not assumed***

Training on a ketogenic approach is not about doing less. It's about doing things better. Performance in boxing depends on how well energy is used, not just how much is available. Understanding the body's energy systems allows you to train with more control, maintain output, and reduce unnecessary fatigue. Strength and conditioning remain essential. When training is structured properly, strength can be maintained and performance can stay consistent.

Most issues come from poor planning, not the approach itself. Carbohydrates can still have a place. Used strategically, they can support high intensity demands without disrupting the overall system. The key is purpose – not habit. Training must be adjusted to match the system. Pushing without structure leads to fatigue and inconsistency. Adjusting intensity, managing volume, and respecting recovery allows performance to stabilise and improve over time. This is not about chasing effort. It's about building efficiency. When training is applied correctly, energy becomes more consistent, recovery improves, and performance becomes more reliable – round after round.

# ROUND 9

# FASTING AS A TOOL

## *Using Fasting to Support Control and Performance*

Fasting and a ketogenic approach are closely connected. Both rely on the same principle – allowing the body to use stored energy more efficiently. When carbohydrate intake is low, the body shifts into ketosis, using fat as a primary fuel source. Fasting supports this process by extending the period where no new energy is coming in, encouraging the body to continue using stored fuel. This is why fasting often feels easier on a ketogenic approach.

When adapted to a keto approach, fasting can be undertaken with energy levels remaining more stable, hunger reduced, and the body more able to tolerate reduced meal frequency. But this does not mean fasting is required. It is a tool – not a rule.

In boxing, performance comes first. Fasting should only be used when it supports training, recovery, and weight management. Used correctly, it can help improve control, simplify nutrition, and support fat loss. Used incorrectly, it can reduce energy, affect performance, and slow recovery. The key is understanding when and how to apply it. Not every phase of training requires fasting. Not every fighter will benefit from it in the same way. It must fit the system – not disrupt it.

In this round, you'll learn:

- how fasting connects with ketosis and a ketogenic approach
- when it can be useful in boxing
- when it should be avoided
- how to apply it in a controlled and practical way

Fasting is not about doing more. It's about using the system more effectively – when the timing is right.

## 9.1 INTERMITTENT FASTING

Intermittent fasting is a structured way of organising when you eat. Unlike the fasting that is undertaken by some groups for religious reasons, it does not entail restricting water, which should still be taken normally. It does not change what you eat. It changes when you eat. Instead of spreading meals across the entire day, food intake is limited to a specific time window.

The most common approach is a 16:8 structure – 16 hours without food, followed by an 8-hour eating window. Other models can also be used, depending on the individual and the situation:

- 12/12 – a more basic and easier starting point
- 14/10 – a gradual step into fasting
- 18/6 – a tighter eating window for more advanced use

The approach should match your training demands and lifestyle. During the fasting period, the body is not digesting food. This allows it to rely more on stored energy, particularly fat. On a ketogenic approach, this process becomes more efficient, as the body is already adapted to using fat as a primary fuel source. Energy levels often remain stable. There are fewer spikes and drops compared to frequent eating patterns, and hunger becomes more manageable over time. However, intermittent fasting is not about skipping meals randomly. It needs to be structured around training and recovery. If applied incorrectly, it can lead to:

- low energy during sessions
- poor recovery
- reduced performance

The timing of the eating window matters. Training should be supported by proper nutrition, and fasting should not interfere with key sessions or preparation. For some fighters, intermittent fasting can simplify their routine and improve control over food intake. For others, it may not be suitable – especially during periods of high training demand. It is not a requirement. It is an option. Used correctly, it can support the system. Used without structure, it can work against it.

***Coach's Insight:*** *You don't need the most aggressive approach – you need the one you can apply consistently.*

## 9.2 FASTING AND KETOSIS

Fasting and ketosis work in the same direction. Both shift

the body away from relying on constant food intake and towards using stored energy more efficiently.

When you follow a ketogenic approach, carbohydrate intake is already low. This reduces glycogen stores and encourages the body to produce ketones from fat. Fasting extends this process. With no incoming food, insulin levels remain low, and the body continues to use fat as a primary fuel source. This can increase the production of ketones and strengthen the body's ability to stay in a fat-adapted state.

This is why fasting often feels easier on keto. Instead of experiencing sharp drops in energy, the body has a more stable fuel supply. Hunger becomes more manageable, and energy levels remain more consistent.

However, more is not always better. Longer fasting does not automatically mean better results. If fasting is pushed too far, it can lead to:

- reduced training performance
- slower recovery
- increased fatigue

The goal is not to stay in a deeper state of ketosis at all times. The goal is to support performance while maintaining control over energy and body weight. Fasting should work with the system – not against it. Used correctly, it can reinforce ketosis and improve consistency. Used excessively, it can create unnecessary stress on the body.

***Coach's Insight:*** *Just because you* can *fast longer doesn't mean you should. Use it to support performance – not to test your limits.*

## 9.3 WHEN FASTING WORKS

Fasting works best when it supports the overall plan – not when it interferes with it. It can be useful during periods where the focus is on:

- improving body composition
- maintaining weight
- simplifying daily structure

In these situations, fasting can help create control. Fewer meals can reduce unnecessary snacking, improve consistency, and make it easier to manage overall intake without constant tracking. On a ketogenic approach, this becomes more natural.

Stable energy levels and reduced hunger make it easier to go longer periods without food, without feeling drained or distracted. Fasting can also work well on lighter training days. When the physical demand is lower, the body can manage longer periods without food while still maintaining energy and focus.

However, timing matters. Fasting should not compromise key sessions. On days where intensity is high – such as sparring, hard conditioning, or heavy strength work – the body needs support. In these cases, restricting food too much can reduce performance and slow recovery.

Fasting is also more effective when it is consistent. Using it as a regular structure is more beneficial than applying it randomly without a clear reason. The goal is not to eat less. It's to create better control over when and how you eat. Used at the right time, fasting can support the system. Used at the wrong time, it can limit it.

***Coach's Insight:*** *Use fasting when it makes things easier. Not when it makes training harder.*

## 9.4 WHEN TO AVOID FASTING

Fasting is not always the right tool. There are times when it can work against performance instead of supporting it.

Fasting risks differ significantly between sexes due to metabolic and hormonal variations, with women generally experiencing higher sensitivity to fasting-induced stress. Studies indicate that while women metabolise more fat during fasting, they may also face greater disruption to energy, reproductive hormone changes, and higher stress responses.

Fasting risks also differ depending on the phase of training. During periods of high training demand, the body needs regular fuel. Hard sparring, intense conditioning, and heavy strength sessions place significant stress on the system. In these situations, restricting food for long periods can lead to:

- low energy
- reduced output
- slower recovery

This affects not just the session itself, but everything that follows. Fasting should also be avoided when recovery is a priority. After demanding sessions, the body needs nutrients to repair and rebuild. Delaying food intake too long can slow this process and reduce the quality of recovery.

Another situation to be careful with is fight week. At this stage, the goal is control and stability. Introducing or increasing fasting during this time can create unnecessary stress and make weight management less predictable.

Fasting may also not suit every individual. Some fighters respond well to it. Others may experience low energy, poor focus, or inconsistent performance. This needs to be recognised and respected. The key is flexibility. Fasting is not something that must be followed at all times. It should be applied when it supports training – and removed when it does not. Performance always comes first.

---

***Coach's Insight:*** *If fasting is hurting your training, it's not helping your progress. Use it when it fits – not when it forces problems.*

---

**SUMMARY:** ***Use fasting with purpose***

Fasting and a ketogenic approach work in the same direction. Both support the body's ability to use stored energy more efficiently and maintain stable fuel supply through ketosis. This is why fasting often feels easier on keto. Energy is more consistent, hunger is reduced, and the body is less dependent on frequent meals. But fasting is not required. It is a tool. Used correctly, it can help improve control, simplify nutrition, and support weight management. Used incorrectly, it can reduce performance, slow recovery, and create unnecessary stress. Fasting works best when:

- training demand is lower
- structure and consistency are needed
- it supports overall control

It should be avoided when:

- training intensity is high
- recovery is a priority
- it negatively affects performance

There is no single method that works for everyone. The key is understanding when to apply it and when to step back. Fasting is not about doing more. It's about using the system more effectively – at the right time.

# ROUND 10

# WEIGH-IN STRATEGY

## *Final Preparation Without Panic*

The boxer will not fight unless they make weight at the weigh-in. For boxers this can make fight week a time of extraordinary mental and physical stress, as they battle with the scales. Most mistakes happen here. Fighters leave things too late, rely on extreme methods, or try to force the weight down in the final days. This leads to

- unhealthy weight loss methods
- fatigue
- poor training quality
- increased stress
- reduced performance

This is not discipline. It's poor planning.

Fight week should be where everything comes together. This is not the time to experiment, panic, or make drastic changes. It's the final stage of preparation – where control matters more than effort.

In this round, you'll learn:

- how to manage the final stage of weight control
- how to approach water and electrolyte balance
- how to avoid common fight week mistakes
- how to stay sharp and in control

Fight week should not be about suffering. It should be about precision.

## 10.1 FINAL WEIGHT MANAGEMENT

By fight week, most of the work should already be done. Weight should be at or close to target, and the body should not be under extreme stress. This is not the time to try and lose large amounts of weight. The goal is to make small, controlled adjustments – not drastic changes. When weight has been managed properly throughout camp, the final stage becomes predictable. The body responds better, energy remains stable, and performance is not compromised. Final weight management should focus on control. Small reductions can come from:

- slight adjustments in food intake
- managing hydration carefully
- reducing unnecessary variables

Nothing extreme is required. The key is to stay consistent. No sudden changes. No panic decisions. No unnecessary stress. Making weight should feel manageable. Not desperate. The goal is simple: Arrive at the weigh-in in control.

***Coach's Insight:*** *If you're trying to lose kilos in fight week, the mistake happened earlier. Fight week is for control – not correction.*

## 10.2 AVOIDING PANIC

Last minute panic is one of the biggest problems in fight week. It leads to rushed decisions, extreme methods, and unhealthy stress on the body. When a fighter is over their target in fight week, the reaction is often to:

- cut more food
- cut more water
- add extra sessions
- use extreme methods

This cycle leads to poor decisions and unstable performance. This makes things worse for any boxer, but for a boxer on keto it may be dangerous. The boxer on keto needs a different strategy to avoid panic.

Fight week should feel calm. Focused. Controlled.

***Coach's Insight:*** *The scale doesn't control you. Stick to the plan – not your emotions.*

## 10.3 WATER AND SODIUM

Boxers following an ordinary, carbohydrate-based diet are typically carrying up to 5 kilos of water, stabilised by significant sodium reserves, as part of the system that manages glycogen. To make weight, they typically seek to lose the weight of this water by restricting both fluids and sodium before weigh-in and by "sweating it out" with high intensity exercise. The resulting dehydration – typically followed by chaotic rehydration immediately before the fight – will have damaging effects on their fitness and may therefore be counterproductive.

- dehydration places much stress on the body
- mental sharpness may be lost
- physical performance may be unpredictable
- they face the fight with their metabolism in a state of chaos and in need of recovery

Those extreme last-minute methods are damaging, but in the case of a boxer on an ordinary diet they may allow a substantial weight loss to be achieved without endangering long term health.

*This is not the case with boxers on keto.*

Boxers on keto are not carrying that extra water and sodium: they will have lost most of it at the start of transition, when they moved from glycogen to ketones as their primary source of fuel. That water can't be lost twice, so dehydration is not a safe way of making weight drop in fight week.

Boxers on keto should therefore expect to make only very minor changes to their weight as the weigh-in approaches. Their weight should already be under control.

***Coach's Insight:*** *Boxers on keto shouldn't need to dehydrate before a fight, and should not attempt to do so.*

## 10.4 WEIGH-IN STRATEGY

Making weight is not just about hitting a number on a day. It's about a journey that started long before.

For keto boxers, the battle to make weight should have been fought during camp, in a controlled and systematic way. In the final 24 hours, only tiny adjustments should be needed. These should be minimal and planned, not extreme or rushed. If large cuts are still required at this point, the process has not been managed properly.

A few ounces can be crucial however, and a few small adjustments such as the following may allow a boxer to lose key ounces in the last few days before weigh-in, without compromising either their health or their performance:

- In the final two to three days, no additional carbohydrates – keep to a basic 50 grams
- Light meals only in the last 48 hours
- No extra salt in the final 24 hours
- Take only sips of water in the final 12 hours

These measures will result in a small loss of water which should feel steady and predictable – not rushed or forced. Used correctly, this can help you make weight while staying in control. Water and sodium are not the enemy. They are essential tools.

---

***Coach's Insight:*** *Making weight means nothing if you can't perform after it. Arrive ready – not just lighter.*

---

**SUMMARY:** ***Control the process, don't chase the scale***

Fight week is not the time to fix mistakes. It's the time to execute what has already been planned. When the work has been done properly throughout camp, only small adjustments are needed – not drastic changes.

Panic is one of the biggest risks. Reacting emotionally to the scale often leads to extreme decisions that make the situation worse.

Fight week should feel calm. Controlled. Purposeful. When the process is managed correctly, making weight becomes part of preparation – not a fight in itself.

The weigh-in is not the finish line. It's where preparation moves into execution.

# ROUND 11

# AFTER THE WEIGH-IN

## *Calm Not Chaos*

Many fighters focus everything on the weigh-in – then undo it within hours. Desperate preparation for weigh-in is followed by chaotic rehydration and uncontrolled eating, which can leave them feeling heavy, slow, and flat on fight day. Fluids are unstable, electrolytes unbalanced, energy systems out of kilter. This is where fights are often lost before they begin.

Don't go there. The boxer on keto should aim to use the last few days in fine tuning their body ready for the fight – not recovering from desperate measures.

## 11.1 FUELLING FOR THE FIGHT

The keto boxer should not have entered the weigh-in starved and dehydrated, so after the weigh-in only minor changes to nutrition and hydration should be needed to restore proper balance. The last few days can therefore be spent achieving the ideal state for the fight.

Nutrition after the weigh-in is not about eating as much as you want – it's about supporting performance. When weight has been managed properly, the body does not need to be rebuilt. It needs to be supported. The goal is to provide the right nutrients, in the right amounts, at the right time, so the body can perform as intended. Food should be easy to digest and purposeful. The focus is on how the body responds, not just how much is consumed.

Protein supports muscle repair and recovery, helping the body prepare for the demands ahead. Fats provide a steady and reliable source of energy, supporting stability without sharp fluctuations. If carbohydrates are used, they should be controlled and timed around performance demands. They can support higher-intensity efforts by contributing to glycogen availability, but excessive intake can lead to unstable energy, digestive discomfort, and unnecessary weight fluctuations.

The key is balance. Spacing meals over time allows nutrients to be absorbed more effectively. Energy levels rise gradually and remain stable, rather than peaking and crashing. This supports consistent output, clearer thinking, and better control going into competition. On a ketogenic approach, this process can remain more controlled. There is less reliance on carbohydrate intake, and energy can be supported without extreme swings. This often results in a more stable physical and mental state. Fuelling at this stage is not a reward for making weight. It is part of preparation. Every decision should support performance.

***Coach's Insight:*** *Don't let hunger control your decisions. Eat with purpose – not emotion.*

## 11.2 AVOIDING THE BINGE

After the weigh-in, the urge to eat more than needed can still be strong. Mentally, it feels like the hard part is done. This is where control can slip. Even when food has been managed properly throughout the process, the body is still sensitive to how intake is handled at this stage. Eating excessively or too quickly may feel satisfying in the moment, but it can lead to:

- bloating
- sluggishness
- poor digestion
- unstable energy levels

Instead of feeling prepared, you can end up feeling heavy and uncomfortable. The body does not need to be overloaded. It needs to be supported. Large, unstructured intake creates unnecessary stress rather than improving readiness.

Sudden increases in food – especially without control – can also disrupt energy balance. Levels may rise quickly, then drop, making performance feel inconsistent. Control is key. Refuelling should remain gradual, structured, and consistent. Meals should be spaced, portions controlled, and choices purposeful. This is not about restriction. It's about maintaining discipline at the point where many fighters lose it. The goal is not to feel full. The goal is to feel ready.

***Coach's Insight:*** *The fight isn't over at the weigh-in. Stay disciplined when it matters most.*

## 11.3 FIGHT READINESS

After the weigh-in, the focus shifts to performance. The goal is simple: Make sure the body is in a state where it can perform at its best, physically and mentally.

The period between the weigh-in and the fight should not be left to chance. In amateur boxing, fighters compete only hours after weighing in, meaning hydration and refuelling must be controlled carefully and efficiently.

In professional boxing, there is more time between weigh-in and the fight (often 24-36 hours) but fuelling still needs to remain controlled rather than excessive.

This stage is not just physical. Mental state also matters. Overthinking, stress, frustration, or emotional highs and lows can affect performance just as much as physical fatigue. The aim is to stay calm, focused and controlled.

Activity during these final hours should be purposeful. Rest is important, but that does not mean doing nothing. Light movement, staying loose and mobility work can help the body to stay ready without creating unnecessary fatigue.

On a ketogenic approach, this period will feel more stable if the process has been managed correctly. There are usually fewer energy swings, more controlled hunger levels, and steadier mental state.

> ***Coach's Insight:*** *You don't need to feel perfect. You need to feel ready to perform.*

**SUMMARY:** ***Prepare to perform***

After the weigh-in, the focus should shift from making weight to preparing the body and mind for performance. Many fighters damage performance by binge eating, overhydrating, or making desperate last-minute changes, leaving themselves heavy, sluggish, and unstable on fight day. A properly managed ketogenic approach helps avoid this chaos by keeping hydration, electrolytes, and energy levels more controlled throughout the process.

Post weigh-in nutrition should be purposeful – not emotional. Meals should be easy to digest, and focused on maintaining stable energy rather than creating spikes and crashes.

Discipline remains essential after the weigh-in. The goal is to feel ready – not full. Alongside physical preparation, staying calm, focused, mobile, and mentally controlled is equally important for peak fight readiness.

# ROUND 12

# LONG-TERM CONTROL

## *Sustaining Performance Beyond the Fight*

For good or ill, the fight is over. And after every fight except the last, the boxer must pick themselves up and begin the rest of their career. A once-off result may be glorious or heart-breaking, but long-term control is what matters. Many fighters can make weight once. Few can do it consistently without damaging performance. That's the difference between a method and a system.

This book is not about quick fixes or extreme approaches. It's about building a way of managing nutrition, weight, and performance that works over time – not just for one fight.

A ketogenic approach, when applied properly, offers structure and stability. It helps reduce reliance on last-minute weight cuts, improves consistency, and allows fighters to stay closer to their natural fighting weight. But the real value is not just in the method. It's in the understanding.

When you understand how your body works, you stop reacting and start controlling the process. You don't need extreme diets. You don't need drastic cuts.

You don't need to repeat the same mistakes. You build consistency. You make better decisions. You stay in control. In this final round, the focus shifts beyond individual fights.

You'll learn how to:

- manage weight across seasons
- avoid rebound and unnecessary fluctuations
- maintain performance over time
- build a sustainable approach to nutrition

This is where everything comes together. Not just for one fight. But for your entire career and your life beyond it.

## 12.1 METABOLIC FLEXIBILITY

Metabolic flexibility is the ability of the body to use different fuel sources efficiently. It means being able to switch between using carbohydrates and fats depending on the situation.

Most fighters rely heavily on carbohydrates. They are used to frequent eating, quick energy, and constant refuelling. When that system is disrupted, energy drops quickly.

A more flexible system changes this. When the body is adapted to using fat as a primary fuel source, it becomes less dependent on constant intake.

Energy becomes more stable, and the body can perform effectively even when food is not immediately available. This does not mean carbohydrates are useless. It means they are no longer the only option. A metabolically flexible fighter can:

- maintain energy over longer periods

- recover more efficiently
- adapt to different training demands
- manage weight with greater control

This is where a ketogenic approach plays a key role.

By reducing reliance on carbohydrates, the body becomes more efficient at using fat. Over time, this improves the ability to switch between fuel sources when needed. This creates more control. Instead of reacting to energy drops, the body can maintain output and adjust more smoothly.

Metabolic flexibility is not built in a day. It comes from consistent application of the system, proper training, and structured nutrition. The result is a more stable, adaptable, and efficient athlete.

> ***Coach's Insight**: Don't rely on one fuel source. The more options your body has, the more control you have.*

## 12.2 OFF-SEASON CONTROL

The off-season is where many unseen mistakes happen. There is no fight date, no pressure from the scale, and less structure in daily routine. This often leads to a loss of control.

Weight increases. Habits slip. The gap between walking weight and fighting weight grows.

This creates problems later. The bigger the gap, the harder the cut. The harder the cut, the greater the stress on the body. The cycle repeats.

Off-season is not a time to lose discipline.

It's a time to build control. This does not mean staying in fight condition all year. It means staying within a manageable range. Close enough that preparation does not require extreme measures. On a ketogenic approach, this becomes easier to manage. Stable energy levels and reduced cravings can help maintain consistency without constant restriction. There is less need for large swings in food intake and body weight.

The goal is simple: Avoid drifting too far away.

Small fluctuations are normal. Loss of control is not. Managing the off-season properly makes everything easier when preparation begins again. Less stress.

Less drastic changes. Better performance.

> ***Coach's Insight:*** *What you do between fights decides how hard the next one will be. Stay in control – even when there's no pressure.*

## 12.3 AVOIDING REBOUND

Rebound weight gain is one of the most common problems

in boxing. After a fight, structure drops. Training intensity often decreases, food intake increases, and discipline fades. The body, coming out of restriction and stress, responds quickly. Weight goes up – often faster than expected. This is not just about eating more. It's a combination of:

- increased food intake
- fluid retention returning
- reduced activity
- loss of routine

The result is a rapid increase in body weight, often beyond the original starting point. This creates a bigger problem for the next camp. More weight to lose.

More stress on the body. More extreme measures needed. The cycle repeats.

Avoiding rebound starts with awareness. After the fight, the goal is not to stay restricted – but to stay controlled. Gradually increasing food intake, maintaining some structure in training, and keeping basic habits in place helps stabilise the body.

On a ketogenic approach, rebound can be reduced. There is less extreme fluctuation in water weight, and appetite tends to be more controlled. This makes it easier to avoid large swings in body weight. But discipline still matters. The system helps – but it does not replace control. The aim is not perfection. It's stability. Small increases are normal. Large, uncontrolled rebounds are not. Managing this phase properly makes the next preparation easier, healthier, and more effective.

---

***Coach's Insight:*** *The fight is over – but the process isn't. Stay in control, or you'll pay for it next time.*

---

## 12.4 CONSISTENCY

Consistency is what holds everything together. Not extreme diets. Not short-term effort. Not one perfect camp. Consistency. The best results in boxing don't come from doing things perfectly for a few weeks. They come from doing the right things, over and over again. Managing weight, nutrition, hydration, and training is not a one-time task. It's an ongoing process. Small, consistent actions lead to:

- ✓ stable body weight
- ✓ better energy levels
- ✓ improved recovery
- ✓ more reliable performance

Inconsistent habits lead to the opposite. Large weight fluctuations. Unpredictable energy. More stress during preparation.

This is where many fighters struggle. They switch between extremes – strict during camp, uncontrolled outside of it. That cycle makes everything harder. A structured approach breaks that pattern. On a ketogenic approach, consistency becomes easier to maintain. Stable energy, reduced cravings, and better control over intake support long-term habits without constant restriction.

But the system only works if it is applied consistently. Not perfectly. Consistently. The goal is not to be strict all the time. It's to stay in control most of the time. That is what builds long-term performance.

> ***Coach's Insight:*** *You don't need to be perfect. You need to be consistent. That's what separates short-term results from long-term success.*

**SUMMARY:** ***Control over time***

Long-term performance is built on control. Not extreme methods. Not last-minute fixes. Not short-term results. Control. Metabolic flexibility allows the body to use energy more efficiently and adapt to different demands. It reduces reliance on constant refuelling and creates more stable performance.

Managing the off-season prevents unnecessary weight gain and reduces the need for drastic cuts. Staying within a controlled range makes preparation easier and less stressful. Avoiding rebound is essential. Rapid weight gain after a fight creates bigger problems for the next camp. Maintaining structure helps keep the body stable and ready.

Consistency holds everything together. Small, repeated actions lead to better energy, better recovery, and more reliable performance over time. This is not about perfection. It's about staying in control.

When the system is applied consistently, weight becomes easier to manage, performance becomes more stable, and preparation becomes more predictable. This is how fighters improve – not just for one fight, but for their entire career.

*You don't win on the scale. You win in the ring.*

*And how you manage your body decides which version of you shows up.*

*Stay in control – Train smart.*

*Perform when it matters.*

## GLOSSARY OF KEY TERMS

Clear and practical explanations to help you better understand weight management and nutrition.

---

**Adaptation**
The process where the body adjusts to a new way of eating or training. In keto, this means learning to use fat and ketones instead of carbohydrates for energy.

---

**Body Composition**
The ratio of fat, muscle, and other tissues in the body. In boxing, the goal is to reduce body fat while maintaining strength and muscle.

---

**Calorie Deficit**
When you consume fewer calories than your body needs, leading to weight loss. If managed poorly, it can also reduce energy and performance.

---

**Carbohydrates**
A quick source of energy found in foods like rice, bread, fruit, and sugar. Mainly used for high-intensity efforts such as fast combinations and explosive movements.

---

**Dehydration**

A state where the body loses more fluid than it takes in. This reduces performance, slows reactions, and increases fatigue.

---

**Electrolytes**
Minerals such as sodium, potassium, and magnesium that control hydration, muscle contraction, and nerve function. Essential for performance, especially on a low-carb or ketogenic approach.

---

**Energy Systems**
The different ways the body produces energy depending on the demands of activity. Fast systems rely more on carbohydrates, while longer efforts rely more on fat.

---

**Fat Adaptation**
The process of becoming efficient at using fat as the main fuel source. Leads to more stable energy and less reliance on frequent refuelling.

---

**Fats**
A long-lasting source of energy. In a ketogenic approach, fats become the primary fuel for training, recovery, and overall performance.

---

**Glycogen**

The stored form of carbohydrates found in muscles and the liver. It provides quick energy for high-intensity actionsbut is limited and runs out quickly.

---

**Insulin**

A hormone that controls blood sugar and energy storage. Lower levels support fat use as fuel and help reduce energy spikes and crashes.

---

**Ketones**

Energy molecules produced from fat in the liver when carbohydrate intake is low. Used by the brain and muscles as an alternative fuel source.

---

**Ketosis**

A metabolic state where the body uses fat and ketones instead of carbohydrates as its main energy source.

---

**Keto Adaptation (Keto Flu)**

The early phase of switching to a ketogenic approach, where energy may feel low and unstable due to fluid, electrolyte, and fuel changes. Temporary if managed properly.

---

**Macronutrients**

The three main components of food: protein, fats, and carbohydrates. Each plays a key role in energy, recovery, and performance.

---

**Metabolic Adaptation**
The body's response to reduced calorie intake, where it lowers energy use to conserve fuel. This can slow fat loss and affect performance.

---

**Protein**
A nutrient used to repair and rebuild muscle. Essential for recovery, maintaining strength, and protecting muscle during weight loss.

---

**Recovery**
The process where the body repairs and rebuilds after training. Proper nutrition, hydration, and rest are essential for improvement.

---

**Satiety**
The feeling of fullness after eating. Higher satiety helps control hunger and prevents overeating.

---

**Thermic Effect of Food**
The energy the body uses to digest and process food. Protein has a higher thermic effect, meaning the body uses more energy to process it.

---

**Water Balance**

The balance between fluid intake and fluid loss in the body. Critical for maintaining performance, especially during training and weight management.

## REFERENCES

**American College of Sports Medicine (ACSM)** (2007). *Exercise and Fluid Replacement.* Medicine & Science in Sports & Exercise.

**Burke, L.M. and Hawley, J.A.** (2018). *Swifter, higher, stronger: What's on the menu?* Science, 362(6416), pp. 781–787.

**Casa, D.J. et al.** (2010). *National Athletic Trainers' Association Position Statement: Fluid Replacement for Athletes.* Journal of Athletic Training, 45(3), pp. 292–303.

**England Boxing** (2023) *Coaching Framework and Athlete Development Guidance.*

**GB Boxing** (2022). *Performance Pathway and Athlete Development Model.*

**Hall, K.D.** (2012). *Metabolic adaptations to weight loss.* Obesity, 20(1), pp. 1–6.

**McArdle, W.D., Katch, F.I. and Katch, V.L.** (2015). *Exercise Physiology: Nutrition, Energy, and Human Performance.* 8th ed. Philadelphia: Wolters Kluwer.

**Paoli, A., Rubini, A., Volek, J.S. and Grimaldi, K.A.** (2013). *Beyond weight loss: A review of the therapeutic uses of* *very-low-carbohydrate ketogenic diets.* European Journal of Clinical Nutrition, 67(8), pp. 789–796.

**Phillips, S.M. and Van Loon, L.J.C.** (2011). *Dietary protein for athletes: From requirements to optimum adaptation.* Journal of Sports Sciences, 29(sup1), pp. S29–S38.

**UK Sport** (2021). *Performance Nutrition Guidelines for Olympic and Paralympic Sport.*

## EVIDENCE AND FURTHER READING

The principles in this book are informed by established research and guidance in sports nutrition, hydration, and athletic performance.

Key sources include:

- UK Sport – Performance Nutrition Guidelines
- England Boxing – Coaching and Athlete Development Resources
- American College of Sports Medicine (ACSM) – Nutrition & Hydration Position Stands
- International Society of Sports Nutrition (ISSN) – Position on Diets and Performance
- NHS (UK) – Hydration and General Health Guidance
- Sawka et al. (2007) – Exercise and Fluid Replacement
- Casa et al. (2010) – National Athletic Trainers' Association Hydration Guidelines

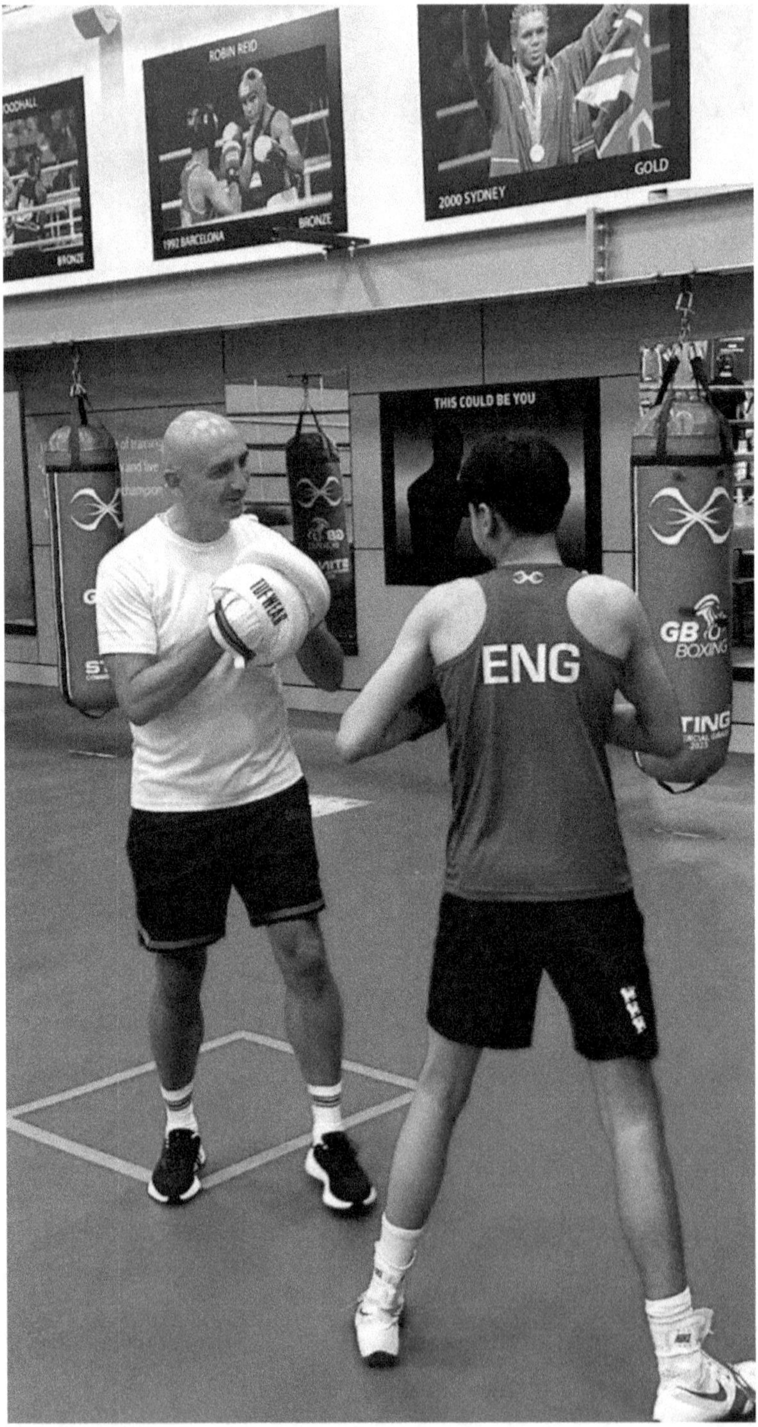
ROBIN REID
1992 BARCELONA
BRONZE
2000 SYDNEY
GOLD
THIS COULD BE YOU
ENG
GB BOXING

## ABOUT THE AUTHOR

Andy Hodges is an England Boxing Level 3 Senior Coach and a BBBofC (British Boxing Board of Control) trainer/second, with over 35 years of experience in boxing and combat sports.

He spent over 16 years competing in kickboxing and boxing at both amateur and professional levels, before moving fully into coaching, athlete development, and education.

His approach combines practical coaching experience with evidence informed principles focused on performance, discipline, and long term athlete development.

He is the founder of Boxing Lab Academy, where he works with boxers of different ages and abilities helping athletes train with clarity, control, and purpose.

**DISCLAIMER**

This book is for educational purposes only and is based on coaching experience and applied practice in boxing and performance. It is not medical advice. Before making changes to diet, hydration, or weight management, consult a qualified professional, especially when preparing for competition. All responsibility for how this information is used remains with the reader.



*For boxers, coaches, and anyone committed to smarter preparation.*

www.ingramcontent.com/pod-product-compliance
Lightning Source LLC
LaVergne TN
LVHW022219200926
848481LV00006B/2026